Naturally,

You Want To Lose Weight—

so why not diet naturally? Lelord Kordel, world-famous health food authority, shows you how, with a simple mixture of cider vinegar, honey, and safflower oil that will not only allow you to lose weight and keep it off, but will increase your vitality and make you feel and look younger.

There are many different ways to diet naturally, and you can select the one that will work best for you. Without living on rice or carrot sticks, you can whip up satisfying meals that burn fat instead of stockpiling it. Learn the eat-your-age way to stay slim, even crash diet (if you must) safely and effectively without loss of energy. Shape up, slim down, and stay that way with organically balanced dieting that really works . . . and works wonders!

SIGNET Books of Special Interest

LELORD KORDEL'S

Secrets
for
Staying Slim

A SIGNET BOOK from
NEW AMERICAN LIBRARY
TIMES MIRROR

Library of Congress Catalog Card Number: 78-136793

*This is an authorized reprint of a hardcover edition published
by G. P. Putnam's Sons. The hardcover edition was published
simultaneously in Canada by Longmans
Canada Limited, Toronto.*

SIGNET TRADEMARK REG. U.S. PAT. OFF. AND FOREIGN COUNTRIES
REGISTERED TRADEMARK—MARCA REGISTRADA
HECHO EN CHICAGO, U.S.A.

SIGNET, SIGNET CLASSICS, SIGNETTE, MENTOR AND PLUME BOOKS
*are published by The New American Library, Inc.,
1301 Avenue of the Americas, New York, New York 10019*

FIRST PRINTING, AUGUST, 1972

3 4 5 6 7 8 9 10 11

PRINTED IN THE UNITED STATES OF AMERICA

TO LORDEEN

my lovely, figure-conscious daughter who, in addition to serving as a part-time "guinea pig," also kept an eagle eye on my busy schedule to make sure I *made* the time to follow my diet program so that the surplus weight I had allowed to accumulate would roll off. And it did!

Contents

1

Are You a Diet Dropout?

As your weight goes up, your life expectancy goes down.
And, if you're among the majority of adults, you either
have a weight problem, have had one, or will have one
sometime in your life.

In a nationwide poll conducted by Alfred Politz Research, Inc., some staggering estimates were produced:

*A total of 58 percent of all adults in America suffer
from obesity in some degree.*

Although women dieters outnumber men (by 72 percent to 28 percent), the Politz poll found that men are
better at sticking to a diet, and generally lose more while
on it than do the women.

The reason? For the most part, men have a much
stronger motivation than women.

It makes a big difference whether you want to lose
weight so you can wear a bikini, or because your doctor
has warned you of the danger of high cholesterol, clogged
arteries, and a possible coronary attack.

Not until a woman is past the menopause does she face
the same risk as a man from heart and artery damage.
Until then, staying on a diet is not a matter of life and
death for her.

She may want to reduce because she thinks that today's
clothes are designed solely for a slender, youthful figure,
which most of them are. Yet it could be that a false
optimism created by the clothing manufacturers themselves is partly responsible for the increasing number of
diet dropouts.

They have developed what one designer calls "a happy

deception—slimming by psychology" that helps convince a woman her dimensions are dwindling when they aren't.

Don't delude yourselves, girls. Although the size of your suits and dresses is shrinking, it doesn't mean that you are. It's all part of the garment makers' "happy deception."

Remember when a size 3 dress was strictly for toddlers?

I thought it still was until I saw a 106-pound grandmother buying one—not for her grandchild, but for herself!

Here is how an award-winning designer, Margit Fellegi, explains it: The size 3 of today was actually a size 8 back in the days when size tags were honest instead of deceptive. And the size 5 you're hoping to diet yourself into would have been a 10 just a few years ago.

"Today's basic pattern measurements are bigger than they were when I started designing 24 years ago," Miss Fellegi says. "The woman's frame is bigger, her shoulders are broader, her entire bone structure is enlarged."

A woman hasn't much incentive to reduce if she thinks she is getting smaller because her dress size is. But sooner or later the diet dropout may find that she must resort to camouflage to hide the figure beginning to burst the seams of a size 12 (actually a 16?).

Isn't that motivation enough for her? It would be for the woman who values her health and vitality, takes pride in her appearance, and wants to keep the romance she has—or get a new one. But not for the chronic diet dropout.

Not as long as she can buy shifts that conceal her shape, wear muumuus at the beach, throw away her tape measure and call the scales a liar. Not as long as she refuses to wake up to reality, see herself as she really is and do something about it.

A few bulges here and there spoil her looks and threaten her lovelife, but not her life. Not yet. At least not as early as a man's life is jeopardized.

Today's doctors are warning their male patients, just as Hippocrates did in his ancient Aphorism No. 44: *"Sudden death is more common in those who are fat than in those who are lean."*

Suppose you're one of the lucky ones who has enough money to buy a new heart if yours gives out?

If you want your luck to last, better keep the one you have in good repair. No matter how much you pay for it, no guarantee goes with a transplant. And no refund is given for those that don't last, even if you were around to collect it.

For centuries, corpulence in a man was admired as a symbol of prosperity. Why not? When food was scarce only the wealthy man could afford what it took to produce a paunch. As his wealth increased, so did his waistline. As for women, his taste ran to what he called "a plump armful," the type immortalized by the artists and authors of his day.

At a time when eighteen-course meals were taken for granted, it was with good reason that the dining room table was known as the groaning board.

During the past hundred or so years we have reduced our meals from eighteen courses to no more than four or six.

What we haven't reduced proportionately is ourselves. Overweight is considered by many authorities as today's Number One public-health problem.

Just a few excess pounds have an unsightly way of settling in all the wrong places. On women it usually forms a bulge in the midriff and heavy, sagging breasts, or pads of fat on the hips and folds of flab you-know-where. More characteristic of men are fleshy jowls and the blob of blubber known as the bay window or potbelly.

Slim-line slacks and skirts require expensive alterations to fit a figure that's out of proportion, whether it's male or female. But these are minor problems compared to those that follow.

As I've said earlier, as your weight goes up, your life expectancy goes down.

You become more vulnerable to diseases of the heart, arteries, liver, and kidneys, all of which can shorten your life. Both men and women who are overweight are more susceptible than thin ones to almost every ailment, including varicose veins, gall-bladder infection, gall stones, and diabetes.

In love or business, the man with a paunch loses his punch.

Personnel agencies agree that being overweight is bad business. Their experience shows that executives who are overweight impair not only their health and initiative but their incomes.

Bernard Willens, vice-president of Robert Half Personnel Agencies, Inc., says, "The difference between the trim, top-dollar man and his overstuffed, lower-paid colleague may be measured at so much per pound, maybe even up to about $1,000 a pound."

The agency claims that fat executives may lose up to $10,000 a year in salary to the lean go-getter who keeps himself physically and mentally fit.

A doctor in San Diego, California, who specializes in the application of diet to overall health warns overweight business men that too much food and drink tends to dull the senses and decrease efficiency. "When a man is from, say, 10 to 30 pounds overweight," says Dr. Roger Lawshe, "potential health problems appear which might well affect his business career."

Among the dangerous conditions in which overweight is a factor, Dr. Lawshe mentioned hardening and thickening of the artery walls and the cerebral blood vessels. When the vessels to the brain are affected, the mind loses its alertness and there may be a progressive decline of mental capacities. Along with it, naturally, goes a decline in income.

According to Dr. Lawshe, if a man lacks the drive or is too lazy to make the effort to take off weight, he is likely to carry the same attitude into his work. And no doubt into his lovelife.

If your butcher and baker are fat you blame it on their occupation, and it doesn't concern you. But if overweight slows down the policeman in your city it could be cause for alarm. Well, Police Chief Jerry V. Wilson isn't going to let that happen in Washington. In August, 1969, he ordered every member of the force to get weighed—with subsequent weigh-ins scheduled regularly every six months.

Overweight Washington policemen now have a strong incentive to get back in shape and stay that way. It was given to them in the form of an ultimatum: reduce or face suspension.

Recent evidence indicates that serious overweight may start at an earlier age than we used to believe. It has been found that our total number of fat cells is established early in life. If you were overfed as a baby, you will have a larger number of fat cells than normal. And that total remains constant as an adult.

When you gain weight, you don't increase the number of your fat cells. You simply fill up the ones you have. As you lose weight your fat cells shrink, but unfortunately they don't disappear. You're stuck with the same number you acquired from eating too many calories as a child.

In children, as in adults, a pattern of overeating conditions the stomach to more food than it requires and creates an abnormal appetite that results in overweight.

Many diet dropouts are victims of a lifetime habit of overeating that has given them an appetite extremely difficult to curb. (Yet it *can* be curbed, as this book will show you.) You see examples of it in the overweight men and women whose main interest seems to be, "When do we eat?"

Another example of early conditioning is the overfed child with an oversupply of fat cells. Unlike other children, he doesn't believe that happiness is a warm puppy. To him it's a hot dog!

Dr. Seymour Halpern, who specializes in both nutrition and medicine, says this of such a child, "Later in life he may have a problem maintaining a sensible weight."

Dr. Halpern calls the discovery concerning fat cells a whole new concept of the physiology of overweight. "This may explain," he says, "why some people are apparently able to eat more than others without weight changes."

So now I suppose some of you will alibi, "It's my fat cells" instead of "It's my glands."

Yet the odds are still about a thousand to one that it's nothing more complicated than your appetite. Even an excessive number of fat cells is no excuse for being fat. Reducing may be more difficult for you, but it isn't impossible.

You must do something about your appetite if you want to lose weight without going hungry.

"But I *do* something about it," you tell me. "I practically starve myself. I go on a crash diet and lose 5 or 6 pounds. The trouble is, as soon as I start eating again I gain them right back."

A starvation diet isn't the answer. I said "lose weight without going hungry," and you can't do that by starving yourself.

Some diets are like a never-ending game of put-'n-take in reverse. You take off a few pounds only to put them back on again. The same 5 or 6 pounds, over and over. Again and *again* and AGAIN.

This off-again, on-again type of reducing is described by

Harvard's Dr. Jean Mayer in words pregnant with meaning. She calls it "the rhythm method of girth control."

You can lose weight quickly on a crash diet or in a steam bath, but it will be mostly liquid weight. And you will gain it back almost immediately, as the head of two great department stores found out.

Bernard Gimbel, a big man with a tremendous appetite, once told his friend Gene Tunney that he figured he had lost about 20,000 pounds in his life.

"I exercise and take a steam bath and lose 5 pounds each time," he said. "But I love to eat, so I put it right back on. I do that at least 200 days a year. One thousand pounds a year for 20 years—that's ten tons over the years."

A leading authority on diet and nutrition, Dr. Norman Joliffe, told of a patient who probably holds the women's record for off-again, on-again dieting. During years of trying one crash diet after another she had lost 500 pounds —and was still overweight.

Dr. Joliffe was gallant enough not to mention the woman's name, but the runner-up for the diet dropout title is a man who doesn't mind admitting it. Martin Lederman, management consultant, world traveler and gourmet, wrote about it in a book called *The Slim Gourmet*.

During 25 years and almost as many different diets he lost a total of 400 pounds—only to eat every one of them back on again. At least he did until he finally became a *reformed* diet dropout. He discovered a way of eating that enabled him to be a slim gourmet instead of a fat one. (See Chapter 11, "Thirty-five Ways to Be a Good Loser" for some of his tips on eating less but enjoying it more.)

You don't have to be a diet dropout. *There is a diet you can stay on without going hungry.*

I found out about it during a recent stay of several months in Greece, where I divided my time between work in Athens and in frequent trips to the mountains.

Searching out the interesting characters among the mountain folk, getting acquainted with them and digging up their almost forgotten folklore was an exciting experience for me.

It was an old Greek mountaineer who told me of a simple diet formula that has kept his people slim, strong and healthy for generations. Many years ago his family had given it to a famous diet dropout of the nineteenth century—Lord Byron, the great poet, adventurer and lover.

The formula was a good one, as I was to find out later, but Byron used poor judgment in following it. In a desperate attempt to shed the fat that spoiled his good looks and slowed down his amorous conquests, he became a dietary eager beaver.

Instead of taking it as directed and making the necessary healthful changes in his eating pattern, Byron went on a starvation diet, eating practically nothing. With little or no food in his stomach, he drank large amounts of one part of the formula while omitting the other two equally important ingredients.

The sad part of the story is that Byron had in his possession a weight-control formula that if properly followed could have slimmed him down with reasonable speed, helped restore his weakened body to health, and perhaps added at least a few more decades to his brief 36 years of life.

Since Lord Byron's time, the formula passed from one generation of Greek mountaineers to another without ever being formally recorded until now.

My own weight seldom varies more than a few pounds, but while I was in Greece I purposely allowed myself to gain some 15 pounds (pounds which I certainly had the intelligence and knowledge to avoid) so I could test the formula on myself before recommending it to others.

How well it worked for me is detailed in another chapter. But I knew that I wouldn't be satisfied until I had proved its effectiveness on persons who have struggled for years with serious problems of overweight.

I wanted to test it on the difficult cases who seemed psychologically incapable of resisting food, the ones with a long history of losing a few pounds and eating them right back on again, those chronic overweights—the diet dropouts.

It wasn't hard to find them. About half the people who come to me for help are diet dropouts who have been told that their obesity is an incurable disease.

Yet by adding Lord Byron's formula to a planned diet, their craving for food was controlled, they reduced to their normal weight, and to their own amazement they *stayed* reduced.

The following chapters will tell what the formula is, how to use it, and why it succeeds when other methods fail.

No matter what you've been told, calories *do* count, especially the *type* of calories you eat. But with this method you don't have to count them.

Instead, you will learn the type of calories that most readily *turn* to fat—and those that *burn* fat.

You will see how a simple, healthful formula that you mix in your own kitchen will aid the fat-burning process, allow you to eat well, yet lose weight and improve your health and vitality at the same time.

Everything in the formula has been recommended many times in my books. For years I have used all of them separately almost every day. The chances are that you have all of the slimming ingredients in your kitchen right now. If not, they are no farther away than your nearest market.

You've heard the old saying, Fight fire with fire. Well, I'd like to paraphrase it to read *Fight fat with food.*

The right kind of food (which you'll learn about later) combined with the formula from the Greek mountains can give you a safe and effective fat-fighting tool.

All you need to make it work for you is the knowledge this book provides and your own determination. With maybe a dollop of positive thinking to help you create a new, slim image of yourself and make it a reality.

Four of the main factors said to cause early aging, especially in women, are overweight, crash diets, the *fear* of aging, and a lack of love. So if you have ever worried about your age, weight, and loveless life, remember this:

You may be a woman that's too young for Medicare— but shape up and you won't be too old for men to care!

2

Formula HOV and What It Can Do for You

To avoid confusion, let me explain that Formula HOV is simply a new, less complicated name for the one mentioned earlier as Lord Byron's or the Greek mountaineer's formula.

My first inclination was to call it the Lord Byron Formula.

The complete formula, taken as directed, would have helped Byron lose weight and protected his nutritional health and balance at the same time.

But as you already know, that wasn't the way he took it.

The legend of Lord Byron still stirs my imagination and evokes memories of poetry, beauty and romance. But, instead of staying with the method that would have reduced him safely and surely, he went on what was one of the first recorded crash diets—and certainly one of the worst.

Because of that it would be misleading to give his name to what I consider one of the best and safest slimming formulas I have ever known. After thinking it over, it seemed to me that it should be given a name that *suggests* a formula. One concise and easy to say. Something short and authentic—maybe an abbreviation.

So I began to think of it in terms of the initials of its three ingredients. Here is what they are, and the equation reached:

HONEY, OIL AND VINEGAR = FORMULA HOV

It sounds deceptively simple, doesn't it? But there is nothing deceptive about what it can do for you.

Turn the words around, give the initials a different meaning, and we have an equation that reads like a promise.

FORMULA HOV = HATED OVERWEIGHT VANISHES

With HOV you don't have to go on a starvation diet to get slim and stay slim. Assuming that you don't have an appetite like Henry VIII, you can eat enough to satisfy it and prevent the hunger pangs that are suffered on most diets. *You can lose weight while eating well and enjoying meals that help you burn fat instead of stockpiling it.*

You will learn which foods you may have in almost unlimited amounts, which ones you may eat in moderation—and those that are off limits except for very rare occasions.

Here is the basic formula of HOV, which can be varied to suit your needs, the occasion or your convenience.

FORMULA HOV

2 tsp. honey
2 tsp. safflower oil
2 tbsp. (1 oz.) cider vinegar

Mix well. Take 3 times a day, about ½ hour before meals.

The Greek mountaineer who gave Byron the formula advised him to make certain changes in his eating pattern which, combined with the honey, oil, and vinegar, would help him control fat and lose the excess weight he had accumulated.

The man laid great emphasis on the values of the naturally fermented vinegar as the main ingredient. Unfortunately, that was the only part of the formula that Byron followed. He went on a starvation diet, drinking inordinate quantities of vinegar and eating nothing but biscuits.

The result was the same as that of the prolonged crash diets of today—Byron lost weight at the expense of his health.

How different were the results in my overweight clients who used the formula with the diet plan I gave them. I saw it succeed time after time in cases where other methods had failed. I saw the "hopeless" cases improve in health as they gradually reduced to their normal weight.

As my own guinea pig, I saw how quickly and easily it enabled me to shed the 15 pounds I had gained so that I might test it on myself.

The next chapter will tell you of several different but equally effective ways of including HOV in your diet, and I have tried them all. But most of the time I simply measure it in a cup, stir it, and take it by the spoonful. To me it's very pleasant tasting, like a honey-flavored French dressing.

If I'm on a tight schedule and know in advance that I'll be having luncheon at my desk I take a small jar of the premeasured formula to the office with me.

The very nature of my work makes it difficult for me to be the guinea pig in any reducing experiment. I'm often invited to speak—and expected to eat—at luncheons, dinners and banquets. My lectures involve considerable traveling and I must have many of my meals on planes and in restaurants, or as a guest in the homes of my sponsors.

But if I manage to take HOV in some form under extremely adverse circumstances, so can you.

There will, of course, be places where you're unable to choose the kind of food necessary to keep your weight down and your vitality up, occasions when it would be rude to refuse what's set before you. I know. It's one of my constant problems. And the best way I know to resolve it is this:

When it's impossible to control *what* you eat, control the *amount*.

No one is going to force you to eat every morsel on your plate. Only an uncontrollable appetite and a lack of willpower can do that. And with HOV included in your

diet you won't need a lot of willpower to curb your
appetite. It does the job for you, so you aren't tempted to
eat too much of the high-carbohydrate, calorie-loaded
foods.

*Yet as I told you, with HOV you don't have to count
calories.*

No longer will you have to do a quick estimate of the
calories in the food on your plate and stop in the middle
of a bite when you've reached your quota for the day.
Neither will you have to get up from the table feeling
hungry, frustrated, irritable, and deprived.

That doesn't mean you can forget about calories or
ignore them completely. You can stop counting them. But
not until you understand how and why you can lose
weight *without* counting them.

You know that a calorie measures energy in terms of
heat, and that it refers to the units of heat, or energy,
which the body gets from its food. Heat given off by the
fuel in a fireplace or furnace is measured in British Ther-
mal Units. Heat given off by the food in you is measured
in calories.

One calorie is the amount of heat required to raise the
temperature of a pint of water to 4 degrees Fahrenheit.
Whether the calorie comes from carbohydrates, proteins,
or fats, it represents the same amount of heat.

But what a difference it makes to you when you're
trying to lose weight.

Food is the fire that warms and invigorates you, the
fuel that keeps you going in high gear. Yet most of you
have seen how one type of fuel burns low, sputters,
smolders, and leaves a residue of ashes while another
burns high and steady with a clean, bright flame.

So it is with the type of calories your body burns for
energy.

Your *basal* metabolism (your heat or energy production, measured in calories) represents the least number of
calories required to maintain vital functions when you're
sitting relaxed at a comfortable room temperature with
your mind, body, and digestion completely at rest.

Women have a slightly lower basal metabolism than
men of the same age, but it gradually decreases in both
sexes as they grow older.

Total metabolism is the total energy expenditure. It

includes that converted into building and repairing tissues, the heat produced by eating, exercising, working, loving, hating, and other emotions, pressures or discomforts that cause tension and restless activity.

The effect of food in raising the metabolism above its basal level is called its *specific dynamic action*. Your metabolism starts to rise about an hour after a meal, reaches its peak in about three hours and by the sixth to eighth hour it drops back down to a fasting level. You can see by that why you should never try to reduce by skipping meals.

You can lose weight faster on the *same amount of food* if it's divided into several smaller meals throughout the day, as reformed breakfast-skippers can testify.

If you've read my other books you know that protein is the food noted for its *specific dynamic action*. Of all foods, protein causes the greatest rise in metabolism. Carbohydrates cause the least.

The person who gains weight easily and seems unable to lose even on an extremely low-calorie diet may be one of the many whose body fails to burn up its carbohydrate calories at a normal rate. When not utilized, these calories pile up rapidly as fat.

Protein calories have just the opposite effect. Their *specific dynamic action* whips up the metabolism and stimulates the body to an increased output of energy that burns up the calories consumed and keeps you from getting fat. When your input and output are equal your weight remains normal, but take in more food than you burn and you will gain. Take in less food than you burn and you create a calorie deficit which causes a weight loss.

Each pound of fat on your body represents 3,500 calories; *to lose a pound requires a deficit of 3,500 calories*. For years the basic law of reducing diets has been this: Cut your calorie intake by 3,500 calories over a given time and within that time you will lose a pound.

The principle itself is sound, and you *can* lose weight at the specified rate, as many iron-willed persons have done.

But do you have the willpower to cut your daily calorie intake by one third? Or to slash 7,000 calories out of your weekly meals for the sake of losing two pounds?

If you can, you will almost certainly lose weight. Slowly, perhaps. But surely and safely.

At least it should be sure . . .

IF you can stay on an extremely low-calorie diet long enough for it to be effective without getting so hungry and discouraged that you give up and join the millions of diet dropouts.

Can you?

And it should be safe . . .

IF you know enough about food values to cut your calories by a third without cutting out the nutrients you must have to prevent the deficiency diseases that can wreck your mental and physical health and age you prematurely.

Do you?

Some years ago I wrote, "Calories are the key to successful reducing." They still are. Yet even then I stressed the fact that the *type* of calories can be more important than the *amount*. I also suggested that persons who gained weight easily had a defective mechanism in their bodies *for handling carbohydrates,* a fact emphasized in all the current low-carbohydrate diets.

And there are many such diets. Some of them are good and some are bad. Some of them have far too much saturated fat—the type of fat that can be dangerous when eaten to excess—and others cut out carbohydrates completely. Some are fairly well balanced and some so wildly unbalanced they seem to shout:

"Lose muscle, lose vital tissue, lose your strength and health—maybe your life—what does it matter as long as you lose weight?"

It matters to me. I feel a strong sense of responsibility for the peop' who read my books and follow my advice, and I cannot recommend any diet that overlooks these vitally important facts:

1. One of the great dangers of an unbalanced reducing diet is the loss of protein which is withdrawn from the body's own muscle and vital organs when not enough is supplied in the daily diet.

2. A low-calorie diet that doesn't have enough excess protein to raise the metabolism and burn stored fat inhibits weight loss and leaves you feeling half starved at the same time. A switch to high-protein meals eases your hunger pangs, boosts your metabolism so that combustion

of fat for energy increases—and you lose weight faster than you did on fewer calories.

3. For health insurance, you should have between 80 and 100 grams of protein a day. As little as 400 calories of meat, fish, poultry, yogurt, cheese, buttermilk, skim milk, or other dairy product will supply about 100 grams. Food values can be measured in calories, but that doesn't mean that meals of the same caloric value are equally effective in a reducing diet. As you have seen, they aren't.

4. On a typical low-calorie diet, fats are usually the first calories to be cut, and some of them should be. But by no means all of them. Neither should they be used as indiscriminately as some of the low-carbohydrate diets permit. With so much conflicting advice, what can a dieter believe?

Believe that the unsaturated vegetable oils (such as the safflower oil in HOV) are essential for your health, and when used in moderation can actually help you lose weight. Believe in restricting the saturated fats in butter and whole milk, in trimming the fat from your meat and omitting gravies and sauces. Do *not* believe in diets that allow you unlimited amounts of fat and all the martinis and whipped cream you want, as some recent ones do.

Believe in the low-carbohydrate fruits and vegetables to supply your body's need for natural sugar and starches. If you have a lot of weight to lose you may have to cut down on them for a while, but *don't* believe in the diets that cut them out entirely.

5. The energy value in a meal depends more on *what* you eat than it does on how *much* you eat. You can get fat while eating comparatively small amounts of one type of food, and grow thin while eating man-sized meals of another. When you know which foods should form the basis of your meals and which ones should be restricted or omitted you can lose weight without counting calories or going hungry.

What you will learn to do is to make every calorie count.

With HOV you will not cut out any foods except those which you should omit for the sake of your health, whether you want to lose weight or not.

You will make protein the mainstay of your diet, and you will learn to choose the *type* and *amount* of carbohydrates and fats that are right for you.

What HOV Can Do for You

HOV and the other recommendations in this book can result in a weight loss when other methods have failed, or when you have never been able to stay on a diet before. In some cases the weight loss will be slow, but steady. In others, surprisingly rapid.

Unlike other diets, as you lose pounds with HOV you will also lose that tired, dragged-out feeling and gain new energy and zest for living.

You will feel and look younger. If you are middle-aged or older, many of the signs of age will diminish.

HOV improves a dry, prematurely wrinkled skin, helps it regain some of its moisture and take on a more youthful smoothness and glow.

As fat, sluggishness, and fatigue disappear you can expect your personality to grow more vibrant and your physical and mental vigor to increase.

Most important of all to those of you in your second forty years, the safflower oil in HOV aids in lowering your cholesterol and in reducing your blood fat. This helps delay or prevent atherosclerosis and the damaged arteries that are forerunners of coronary thrombosis and strokes.

With atherosclerosis delayed, your weight back to normal, your tissues and cells renewed and some of your vital organs revitalized, years of dynamic health and happiness can be added to your life.

3

How HOV Helped Me
Lose 15 Pounds Without
Going Hungry

Sitting on the jet that was bringing me back to America from Greece, I felt a fatigue and drowsiness that were unusual for me. Except for the "jet lag" caused by the difference in time when traveling from one part of the world to another, I hardly know what it is to be tired.

Now I was beginning to find out what it was like.

There was an uncomfortable fullness in my abdomen and an unaccustomed lethargy was inching its way through my body and mind. Leaning forward for a magazine, I noticed that my trousers were tight around my waist, and I felt like loosening my belt another notch.

They were the same size suit and belt that I had worn for years, but now both seemed too small for me. A careless cleaner could have shrunk the suit since I last wore it, I thought. But how was it possible for a leather belt to shrink an inch or two just hanging in the closet?

No, the suit and belt hadn't shrunk. I had expanded. I had done so deliberately for my experiment, but . . .

The full impact of it hadn't hit me until I began to evaluate myself and compare the way I usually looked and felt with my present condition. My last weeks in Greece had been busy ones. With other things on my mind, I had little time to think of the results of my overeating until I stepped on the scales the morning I left.

They registered 190 pounds: 15 pounds above my normal weight!

On my six-foot frame, 15 pounds are not as conspicuous as they would be on a shorter person. As the pounds were accumulating nobody seemed to notice them. Hospitable Greek friends kept inviting me to dinner, and my hostesses were delighted to see me break a precedent and take the second helpings and the rich desserts they urged upon me. Yet as I gained, nobody poked me in the ribs and said, "Putting on a little weight, aren't you?"

At the time I remember thinking that I didn't look or feel much different. Knowing that an extra 15 pounds is more weight than a man can safely carry (especially one in his second forty years), I had every reason to believe that it wouldn't affect me seriously.

Lecithin is one of my daily "musts," and as a protective measure during my food binge I doubled the usual intake. Lecithin's emulsifying action helps prevent excess fats in the diet from causing fatty deposits in the arteries and around the heart. Because of that, and because my overweight was of short duration and not excessive, I had no fear of the heart and artery damage that results in other cases.

My health is and always has been excellent. What could I lose—except the pounds that I intended to start taking off as soon as I arrived home?

I knew there was nothing wrong with me that a change of diet wouldn't remedy. But the exhaustion and discomfort continued.

A physical and mental inertia seemed to be weighing me down. Slowing me down, draining my energy.

In theory, I knew what it was like to drag through life carrying 15 or 20 excess pounds. Like carrying a heavy suitcase that you couldn't put down. Now I was experiencing it personally.

I had seen how friends and clients who gained weight slowly over the years hardly seemed to notice the decrease in physical and mental vigor that accompanied it. At this moment I was aware that it didn't have to be a slow process, with signs of deterioration marking the way. It could happen suddenly, with no advance notice.

It's part of my business to know the capabilities of a slim, healthy body and an alert mind, and of how to keep them that way. Yet it's possible for a man to be too busy to realize that he's slipping until his employer or the family doctor warns him, "Get rid of that dead weight, or else . . . !"

A plane is a good place to take stock of one's self, and that's what I was doing. Or at least I was until thoughts of food intruded. I had eaten my usual hearty, high-protein breakfast, but I was hungry. It must be almost time for luncheon, I thought, and glanced at my watch. It was only 10:30 A.M. Just two hours since I had eaten, so there was no reason for me to feel hungry. Yet the more I thought about food the worse it got. It wasn't until the pangs increased that I recognized it for what it was—a gnawing, insistent craving for something sweet!

Is It Hunger—or Appetite?

Although a craving for sweets is one of the symptoms of low blood sugar, that was not my problem. What had happened to me was this:

After a lifetime of healthful eating, a few weeks of overindulgence had put my appestat out of balance.

Appestat, as most of you know, is a word coined by Dr. Norman Joliffe for the automatic weight-regulating mechanism that operates through the appetite.

This cooperative little gadget is located in the hypothalamus, which is in a vital area of the brain near the pituitary gland.

A normal appestat automatically adjusts your appetite to meet your energy requirements, and you maintain your normal weight.

But just as the thermostat that regulates the heat in your home can be set either too high or too low, so can your appestat. If you overeat just once in a while, the normal appestat will adjust so you eat less at the next meal. You won't feel as hungry as usual, and may say, "I don't know why, but I haven't much appetite." Maybe *you* don't know why, but your appestat does.

It's when you repeatedly overeat that you condition your appestat to such a high level that you can no longer be satisfied with average amounts of food.

Overeating doesn't register on the conscious mind until satiety has been reached. You will hardly be aware that it's taking more and more food to satisfy you until you discover that inflation has hit your food budget—and your waistline!

"You've stretched your stomach overeating, so it takes more to fill it," says your spouse. Then you start eating less to "shrink your stomach"—and, hopefully, the grocery bill.

But what is often called stretching the stomach is the appestat adjusting itself to a high level, and shrinking, to a low one.

Hunger is the actual *need* for food, which should be satisfied. It occurs only when the stomach is empty and when the blood sugar is low.

Appetite is the *desire* for food, and it can occur even when the stomach is full. Appetite can be triggered by habit, the smell of cooking, the thought or memory of food, or by any of several psychological or social factors.

It's a safe assumption that it's your appetite, not hunger, that makes you overeat. And the permanent way to curb an abnormal appetite is to reset the appestat to normal.

By nature the appestat seems to be conservative. It *likes* to balance the food and energy budget, to equalize the intake of the one and the outgo of the other. It dislikes changes. You have to shake it loose from the status quo with gradual dietary changes. It takes time to reset it either way. But just as repeated overeating turns it up to a high level, so will gradually changing from an excessive food intake to a moderate one lower it to normal.

For best results, take it in easy stages and be consistent about it. Remember that your appestat resists change, so if you want its cooperation don't try to crash-diet it down. It responds better to steady, progressive conditioning.

I can explain in detail how the appestat is conditioned, yet it never occurred to me that mine would get out of balance.

I had seen it happen to others. But to me? Ridiculous!

Mine had been thoroughly conditioned to a normal level during all of my adult life—at least until the past few weeks. It was a dependable, no-nonsense appestat. Too well-trained to get out of control.

But it had.

And there it was, sending me false hunger signals, clamoring for food that I didn't need. Growling and grumbling its dissatisfaction over its change of level, making me especially ravenous for the sweets and starches that had until lately been restricted in my diet.

Why hadn't I mixed up a small jar of formula HOV and brought it with me on the plane? The safflower oil's high satiety value would have curbed my hunger pangs and the honey would have satisfied my craving for something sweet.

When the stewardess came through again I knew what I would have as a substitute—hot tea with lemon and honey.

After the first few sips of tea I felt some of my old energy beginning to return. By the time I finished it my craving for food had vanished. My body felt stronger, lighter. My mind was relaxed and clear. My appestat was apparently satisfied. It was quiet. Its grumbling had stopped.

You think that sounds like an exaggeration? Well, it isn't. There is a scientific reason for it.

Honey enters the bloodstream quickly and is rapidly absorbed, giving the brain the glucose it must have as its source of energy, to provide maximum power and mental efficiency.

Since the days of the Olympic Games of ancient Greece, athletes have eaten honey to increase their mental alertness, renew their endurance, and to speed recovery from fatigue. Many athletic coaches recommend it as a quick energizer for both body and mind.

When luncheon was served I asked for a salad with oil and vinegar instead of dressing, and I ate that first. It was followed by a broiled steak and fresh asparagus. For dessert I had black coffee. That was all.

I watched the other passengers eating potatoes Chantilly, hot rolls and butter, and strawberry tarts with whipped cream, yet I wasn't tempted.

It was, I thought, a triumph for formula HOV.

The honey in the tea and the oil and vinegar on the salad had not been premeasured according to the formula. But whatever the proportions were, they had worked to curb the appetite that had so recently been on a rampage. I felt satisfied.

It would take time to get my appestat completely back to normal, but it was temporarily under control. And so far it seemed incredibly easy.

Formula HOV had passed its first and perhaps its most

difficult test. There would be many others in the days of reducing ahead, but I was ready for them.

Or at least I would be as soon as I worked out the details of my diet program. I took a notebook out of my briefcase and started writing ...

My Basic Principles of Reducing

1. *Formula HOV half an hour before each meal.* When it isn't convenient to take the original formula, substitute a cup of tea with a little honey and a salad with oil and vinegar (as I had just done).

2. *Foods HIGH in protein and LOW in animal fats and carbohydrates* form the basis of the only *safe* method of reducing.

3. *A minimum of three servings a day of the complete high proteins.* Meat is one of the best sources and it doesn't have to be expensive. The cheaper cuts provide as much or more protein and less fat than the more expensive steaks and prime rib. *Choose three or more of the following for your daily meals.*

Beef, veal, lamb, liver (any kind), kidneys or other organ meats; chicken, turkey, fish, eggs and cheese (especially cottage cheese, for its high protein content, and if available, *feta*, a delicious low-fat Greek cheese).

4. *Include liver in your menu at least twice a week and some kind of seafood four or five times a week,* or every day if desired. Two cups of buttermilk, skim milk or yogurt are needed each day to supply calcium. If they are omitted, be sure to substitute a large serving of cottage cheese, or plan on getting a minimum of 1,500 grams of calcium a day from bonemeal, calcium lactate, or dolomite.

5. *Preferred methods of cooking:*

Meat and poultry: Broil, bake or roast. Stainless steel skillets may be used for panbroiling or sautéing without fat if the heat is kept moderate, and chicken may be "fried" in the oven without fat.

Fish: Broil, bake, poach or steam.

Eggs: May be shirred, boiled, baked, poached, mixed with a little skim milk powder and scrambled in a double boiler, or made into an oven-omelette. (Just beat the eggs, season, and pour into a lightly oiled pie pan or skillet, place under the broiler until one side is cooked, fold over and finish cooking to desired doneness.)

6. *Trim all visible fat from meats before cooking, and limit other fats in the diet.* The safflower oil in HOV and the small amount used in cooking provides the fatty acids essential for health and helps balance out the "hidden fats" in even the leanest meat. But it can't balance a conglomeration of butter, cream, whole milk, gravies, rich sauces, and desserts. And neither can you!

7. *Cut down on carbohydrates.* To stay healthy on a reducing diet, the average person should have a minimum of 60 carbohydrate grams a day.

But unless you learn to recognize and avoid the foods highest in carbohydrates you can easily pack away ten or twenty times more than you need without being aware of it . . .

Until you step on the scales!

Low-carbohydrate vegetables and fruits (listed on pages 191-2) and the honey in HOV will provide all the carbohydrate you need.

Avoid anything made with white flour and sugar— muffins, rolls, bread, crackers, pizza, macaroni, spaghetti and almost all desserts are high in carbohydrate.

Bypass such nutritious but carbohydrate-loaded foods as dried beans and peas, lentils, lima beans, corn, cereals and other grain products until you're thin again. Then to *stay* thin, eat them only in moderation. Potatoes (especially sweet potatoes!) must be restricted in the diet of those who convert carbohydrates into fat instead of burning them.

That was one of comedian Sid Caesar's problems, but it didn't keep him from losing 31 pounds. He did it by concentrating on high-protein foods, cutting down on all carbohydrates, and completely cutting out bread and potatoes. He was able to give them up by practicing a method of conditioning that worked for him.

"There is no bread," he told himself repeatedly. "In the whole world there is no bread. And there is only one baked potato. If you can find it *and if it has your name on it,* you can eat it."

8. *Fresh fruits and fruit juices must be limited on the low-carbohydrate diet.*

It hurts me to say that anything as delicious and health-ful as fruit should be limited, but with a few exceptions,

fruits are high in carbohydrates. Ordinarily I'm a great
consumer of fruit, having it for almost every meal and
often for between-meal snacks. Cutting down on it was
the only difficult part of my diet.

Dr. Jeremiah Stamler, director of the Division of Adult
Health and Aging of the Chicago Board of Health, expresses my own enthusiasm for fruit and my reason for
limiting it on a reducing diet when he says, "I *love* fruit. I
can eat as much as two pounds a day, *and that gets to be
a carbohydrate problem.*"

It does indeed.

So until a steady weight loss has been established, limit
fruits to two a day—or three, if you're above average in
height and bone structure, and lead a physically active
life. One should be a citrus fruit, and the other chosen
from the list of those with a low to moderate carbohydrate content.

9. *Eat adequate amounts of allowed foods,* but forget
about second helpings while you're resetting your appestat. After it's back to normal you shouldn't want extra
portions. If you do, go ahead and have them as long as
they're protein—an extra slice of meat or chicken or a
little more cheese or fish.

10. *Don't skip meals.* To burn food for energy instead
of converting it into fat, and to avoid a drop in blood
sugar that causes hunger pangs, eat three meals a day.
And feature protein in all of them.

The metabolism, or energy production, is low upon
arising. Tests made by Harvard's Dr. G. W. Thorn and
his co-workers confirmed that it rises very little after a
meal high in carbohydrates and fats, while after a meal
high in protein it rises steadily and stays high for approximately six hours.

Skipping breakfast—or any other meal—slows down
the metabolism. Dividing your daily food quota into three
or more approximately equal parts keeps it elevated during the active, waking hours, distributing energy-
production and hunger-satisfaction evenly.

A breakfast containing 20 or more grams of protein
steps up the metabolic fires, starting a process that increases the combustion of fat for energy and helps you
lose weight faster.

As one doctor expressed it to an overweight patient,

"You'll live off the fat of your body instead of the fat of the land."

11. *A reducing diet should contain sufficient vitamins and minerals to prevent deficiencies and to insure good health.*

In a recent book, *Vitamins in Health and Disease, a Modern Reappraisal,* Dr. John Marks of Cambridge University does just what the title indicates—gives them a thorough reappraisal. American nutritionists have long been aware that deficiencies have become more prevalent than ever before in an affluent society, and that the nutritional level of people on well-balanced diets can vary from high to an alarming low. Dr. Marks suggests that we start thinking in terms of *optimal* vitamin and mineral values instead of the outdated and inadequate *minimum daily requirement* or *recommended allowance.*

His conclusion is that supplementation to an *optimal intake* would "result in increased performance and reduced levels of illness."

Whenever possible, I believe in getting all the vitamins and minerals you can from fresh fruits, leafy green salads and other green and yellow vegetables. My normal diet includes all of them in abundance. But even on the best possible diet there are so many factors involved that I consider multivitamin and mineral supplements essential to optimum health, so I never miss taking mine.

I recommend the same health insurance for everyone— and *especially* for reducers and others on restricted diets.

12. *Don't get in a diet-rut, or you're buying yourself a return ticket to Dropoutsville and inviting chronic obesity.*

If you tried to continue indefinitely on a crash, fad, or mono diet your sense of taste would soon rebel—and so, I hope, would your common sense.

If you MUST Crash Diet, you'll find the safest ones to use for an emergency in the chapter with that title. But no recommendation or guarantee goes with them. The duration of each should be strictly limited, and you're almost certain to gain back the pounds you lost when you start eating again.

So unless it's a *real* emergency, why bother?

The secret of *permanent* success in reducing is to establish eating habits that you can continue after you've slimmed down.

You can't do it with crash diets, or with those that limit you to only one or two of the three essential food elements. But you *can* if your meals include a variety of your favorite foods, as this plan does.

Only then can you forget it's a diet and look on it as a healthful, enjoyable way of life.

One that will *keep* you slim.

By the time I put my notebook away the plane was circling Kennedy Airport. After a conference with my editor the next day I left for home, where my HOV method of losing weight without going hungry would become daily routine for awhile.

It's a habit of mine to go on a modified fast now and then when I feel that I need it, especially after a period of eating more heavily than usual. Now, following the only actual food binge of my life, the cleansing process of fasting seemed more vital than ever.

The damage done by weeks of bad eating habits had insulted my body, made my appestat mutinous and my stomach grumble in protest.

My first two days at home I ate no solid food. I drank plenty of water, moderate amounts of vegetable and fruit juices and herb tea, and took the HOV formula three times a day.

The subject of fasting is covered in a later chapter, so I won't go into details here except to mention one amazing fact:

Never at any time was I conscious of the twinges of hunger that are customary during the first few hours of fasting. Formula HOV had again proved its value as an appetite appeaser!

How effective a reducing program is for each person depends upon many things, including height, weight, frame, temperament, age, sex, and physical activity.

There is a wide variance between the nutritional needs of any two individuals. And even within one person the needs change under certain conditions, and from year to year. Sometimes from day to day.

The particular portions that will reduce one person may be too much—or too little—for another, and should be scaled up or down accordingly. The meals that slimmed me down would have to be modified to some extent for shorter, less active men (and especially for women!), or I'd get a lot of angry letters about the results.

If a diet is to work for the majority instead of the few, it should not consist of rigid, no-substitution menus that specify to the ounce how much to eat, as some diets do. To be practical and easy to stay on it must suit a variety of tastes, needs—and pocketbooks. It should allow for any reasonable substitution of foods *within the same category.*

On this diet you can swap *one low or medium carbohydrate vegetable or fruit for another* as long as they're on the same list (pages 191-2).

The *complete proteins* can substitute for each other, if you remember to make up any protein deficits on the deal. For example, substituting one egg for a steak would cost you about 15 grams of protein. Two eggs and a few chicken livers scrambled together would even up the trade, so just use judgment in keeping the exchanges fairly equal in protein value.

And that's where the swapping stops.

No other food element can safely substitute for protein. Neither carbohydrates nor fats. Nothing can—except more protein.

Whether you're dieting or not, hard fats are never a safe substitute for liquid vegetable oils. Switch from low carbohydrates to high, and the excess is deposited as fat, setting you up as a target for a killer called *Overweight.*

Within these limits, make whatever substitutions are necessary to adapt a good, basic diet to fit your individual tastes and needs. If a menu calls for steak and your budget says hamburger, listen to your budget.

Basically, the meals that slimmed me down are much the same as those I've always eaten. The same pattern of eating that maintained my weight for years with little or no variation.

But how to *maintain* my weight wasn't the problem now.

It was how to *lose* 15 pounds of it. Safely, permanently—and without going hungry.

Formula HOV solved the problem for me.

During the first week I lost 7 pounds—almost half of what I wanted to lose! After that it dropped to a steady 2½ to 3 pounds a week.

HOV and high-protein meals didn't waste any time getting my appestat under control. In less than a month I lost the entire 15 pounds.

How to Take HOV

As I told you earlier, when I eat at home or at my desk I take HOV "straight" from a premixed jar of the formula.

If I'm eating in a restaurant, I do as I did on the jet from Greece to New York—order tea with honey and a salad with oil and vinegar before the entrée.

One of my clients who lost 32 pounds with the HOV method likes it blended with half a cup of skim milk and a few fresh berries.

Another shakes it vigorously in a jar with buttermilk and a spoonful of carob powder. (It is really delicious!) Those last two mixtures add to your protein and calcium quota and are filling enough to curb the most ravenous appetite.

A five-foot one-inch diet dropout who was 45 pounds overweight and a chronic breakfast skipper told me that she was too "squeamish" in the morning for anything except coffee. In her case, the pre-breakfast HOV was omitted. Instead, she was gradually conditioned to eat a small but high-protein breakfast.

Mixing a "cocktail" of formula HOV and carbonated water with a dash of lemon or lime juice and taking it half an hour before luncheon and dinner kept her from overeating at those meals. For the first time in her life she was able to stay on a diet until she reached her desired weight of 108 pounds.

For a few clients who were "slow burners" and below average in height, cutting the proportions of the formula in half resulted in a faster weight loss.

Whatever your size, metabolism, and tastes are, HOV can be adapted to suit them. (Except, of course, for diabetics and others whose diet prohibits *any* concentrated sweet, even such a healthful one as honey.)

HOV before meals worked for me by keeping me completely satisfied with smaller portions than I normally eat. It can do the same for you.

When I began my diet I expected to make a conscious effort to eat less, but it wasn't necessary. All I did was to see that it supplied me with the essential nutrients so I wouldn't lose weight at the expense of vital tissue. HOV took care of the *amount*, so I automatically cut down.

Almost at once I began to utilize what I ate as efficiently as I ever had, and to burn the excess of stored fat. My body chemistry, thrown out of balance by an unaccustomed food binge, was getting back to normal, and so was my vitality.

During that first week I could almost see the pounds dropping away. But what's more important, I could *feel* the difference it made in me. I had found out what it was like to be overweight, not in theory, but in reality. I had experienced the frustrations and the physical and mental inertia that accompany excess poundage, and I knew how rapidly they could be restored by a change in diet.

Examples of the menus that renewed my vigor as they reduced me are in the chapter that follows.

Are you ready to join me in a healthful, slimming way of life?

Seven Days of Slimming Menus

The menus listed in this chapter are, of course, subject to change—depending on availability, individual taste and budget. In adapting them for your own use, just be guided by the *types* of foods I found useful in my own reducing program. All you do is take it from there.

EVERY DAY

Before each meal
Formula HOV
or
Tea with honey and salad with safflower oil and cider vinegar.

After breakfast
Vitamin-mineral supplement (my choice is "Nutri-Time")
Extra vitamin C (at least 250 mgs)
Other vitamins and supplements as required

Sometime during the day
1 tablespoon lecithin granules dissolved in bouillon, tomato juice or skim milk, or sprinkled on salad or in food

ANYTIME

Midmorning, midafternoon, or whenever desired

Cup of consommé, bouillon or instant vegetable broth
—hot, jellied, or on the rocks

Buttermilk, skim milk or yogurt (up to a pint a day
total intake)

Coffee and tea—especially herb teas, decaffeinated
coffee or coffee substitute (no cream or sugar, but a
little skim milk may be used if desired)

Choice of Eat-All-You-Want Foods and snacks listed in
Chapter 6

FIRST DAY

(Recipes are given in Chapter 14 for dishes marked*)

Breakfast

 ½ grapefruit
 Scrambled eggs with chipped beef and chopped green
  peppers (cooked in lightly oiled pan or double-
  boiler)
 Choice of beverage

Luncheon

 Baked or broiled fish with cottage cheese and chive sauce
 Lettuce, celery, cucumber and watercress salad with to-
  mato French dressing*
 Glass of skim milk or buttermilk

Dinner

 Lean roast beef
 Shredded cabbage, carrot, and bean-sprout salad
 Asparagus
 Fresh pear
 Choice of beverage

SECOND DAY

Breakfast

 1 medium orange
 Sautéed veal kidney and mushrooms
 Choice of beverage

Luncheon

 Broiled hamburger with slice of tomato and onion
 Calico coleslaw*
 Glass of skim milk or buttermilk

Dinner

 Crabmeat cocktail
 Chicken à la Grecque*
 Broccoli
 Artichoke hearts and leafy green salad
 Honeydew and watermelon balls
 Choice of beverage

THIRD DAY

Breakfast

½ small cantaloupe filled with cottage cheese and topped
with yogurt

Coffee Slim (⅔ cup coffee and ⅓ hot skim milk)

Luncheon (at my desk)

Tin of sardines (packed in oil, with excess drained off)

Celery, radishes, and raw cauliflowerets

2 fresh apricots

Choice of beverage

Dinner

Broiled liver with mushrooms

Steamed minted carrots

Mixed green salad

⅔ cup of diced fresh pineapple

Choice of beverage

FOURTH DAY

Breakfast

Fresh strawberries moistened with orange juice

Baked eggs with anchovies*

Wedge of cheese

Choice of beverage

Luncheon

2 all-beef frankfurters

Hungarian sauerkraut*

Cucumber, sliced beet and chicory salad

Glass of buttermilk

Dinner

Braised sweetbreads

Swiss chard (or collard greens) in mock sour cream*

Combination salad

½ fresh papaya

Choice of beverage

FIFTH DAY

Breakfast

½ grapefruit

Cheese omelette

Choice of beverage

Luncheon (at my desk)

Tin of salmon

Raw carrot, cucumber, and zucchini sticks

3 cottage-cheese-and-chive balls (just drain cheese, mix
with chives and shape into balls)

Glass of skim milk or buttermilk

Dinner
>   Lobster Cantonese*
>   Bean sprouts with celery*
>   Cauliflower
>   Mixed green salad
>   Slice of honeydew melon, lightly dusted with ginger
>   Choice of beverage

SIXTH DAY

Breakfast
>   Tangerine
>   Salmon-egg patty with wheat germ*
>   Choice of beverage

Luncheon
>   Skillet-burger loaf*
>   Dilled green bean, celery, and onion ring salad
>   Glass of skim milk or buttermilk

Dinner
>   Lamb shanks Mediterranean*
>   Steamed turnip greens and shredded turnips
>   Tomato and watercress salad
>   Wedge of cheese and ½ sliced apple
>   Choice of beverage

SEVENTH DAY

Breakfast
>   ½ grapefruit
>   Chicken-liver omelette
>   Choice of beverage

Luncheon
>   Tomato bouillon (⅔ cup of bouillon made with cube
>   and ⅓ cup hot tomato juice)
>   Chef's salad with seafood
>   Choice of beverage

Dinner
>   Broiled steak
>   Panned mushrooms
>   Summer squash
>   Romaine, shredded raw spinach and sliced radish salad
>   Fresh raspberries (or other berries in season) topped
>   with yogurt
>   Choice of beverage

"It's not difficult to diet these days," wrote Eleanor C. Wood in the Philadelphia *Sunday Bulletin.* "Just eat what you can afford."

I like steak as well as anybody, but you won't find the
"celebrity diet" of steak and tomatoes three times a day
included in my recommended diet menus. Yes, you can
lose weight on it. But except for celebrities, who can
afford it?

My job is to help reduce *you*, not your bankroll!

At today's prices, steak at every meal, or even every
day, just doesn't fit into the average budget. If you belong
to the vast majority, it would be a question of which gets
thin first—you or your pocketbook.

Eating to beat the pound and inflation at the same time
can be done, but it takes a little planning. To prove it, I
purposely planned most of my own reducing menus and
the recipes in this book around foods that slim you down
while providing the highest amount of protein at a reasonable cost.

These include lean hamburger and any of the other less
expensive cuts of beef, lamb and veal; liver (beef, calf and
chicken), kidney and other organ meats; chicken, turkey,
fish, seafood, eggs and cheese.

Canned salmon, tuna, sardines and dried chipped beef
can be kept at home or in the office for slimming, satisfying meals that are high in protein and low in cost.

I keep a supply on hand for busy-day luncheons when I
have a deadline to meet and must work overtime at my
desk, as I often do. They take so little time to prepare
that the busiest office worker or housewife can do the
same.

The green and combination salads on my diet can be as
varied as the seasons, so no recipes are given for them.
Make them to suit your individual taste, as I do, by
combining several of your favorites from the following
low-carbohydrate list.

Leafy Greens and Raw Vegetables for Salads

Lettuce, romaine, endive (curly and French), escarole,
chicory, young raw spinach, mustard spinach, dandelion,
mustard and turnip greens, lambs quarters, sorrel, bean
sprouts, tampala, watercress, chopped parsley, celery, cucumber, cabbage (green, red, Savoy and Chinese), green
and red peppers, scallions, radishes, leeks, onion rings,
tomatoes, shredded or sliced young beets, carrots, turnips,

zucchini, summer squash, broccoli, cauliflower, raw sliced mushrooms, egg plant, and pimiento strips.

Next to protein, the leafy greens are probably a dieter's best friend. They're high in vitamins and minerals, and the lowest of all vegetables in carbohydrate, so try to have them often, either alone or mixed with other raw vegetables. And if you haven't taken your formula HOV before eating, don't forget to mix your salad with safflower oil and cider vinegar.

Without HOV you might be tempted to overeat, especially of fattening, high-carbohydrate foods.

And when you do, you know what happens to you . . .

X-cess marks the spot.

The next two chapters tell you why HOV can prevent it.

5

Honey to Curb *Hunger,*
Fat to Fight *Fat,*
Vinegar to Cut *Fat*

There is at least one thing that nutritionists and Madison Avenue have in common.

Both agree that there is what's called a "fat time of day," a time when your appetite gets out of control and a craving for food can sabotage your diet.

To a nutritionist, it's any time the blood sugar drops to a low level and the appestat signals "Hunger!" It's the time of day or night that the willpower and appetite clash in a do-or-diet struggle.

To Madison Avenue, it's a time to promote their client's products with such familiar slogans as The Pause that Refreshes, a time for the sales pitch to increase the hunger, thirst, and hopes of a vulnerable target—the United States of Fat America.

It's a time for advertising's very lucrative hard sell.

And lucrative it is. A well-known "reducing" candy still has an enviable sales record, although the firm has had trouble with the Federal Trade Commission for years.

The FTC branded the company's advertising "deceptive," but admitted that "this candy or any other sweet taken shortly before meals might curb the appetite. ..." And a Court of Appeals decision stated in part:

"The facts are plain, it being undisputed that eating candy before meals curbs the appetite, lessens intake of food, and involves no restriction of diet but automatically restrains the desire for food. ..."

"Reducing" candies won't reduce you unless you diet, but they will depress your appetite to some extent, making it easier for you to stay on a diet. And if you're in normal health, they won't cause the severe side effects that some of the drugs used as appetite suppressants have done.

Amphetamines ("pep pills"), digitalis, and thyroid are the drugs most widely used in reducing programs by the self-styled "obesity specialists," or diet doctors.

An article in the *Journal of the American Medical Association* warned against the misuse of amphetamines, saying that it has become "increasingly clear that many physicians have not fully appreciated the inherent dangers in prescribing these medications. . . ."

Isn't it about time they did?

Listen to a description of the results of too much thyroid by a noted gland specialist, Dr. Herman H. Rubin:

"The heart is but one organ of the body that is *living too fast*, burning itself up in a conflagration instead of living at a steady rate. Unless help is given, the heart that is racing to destruction will eventually be damaged beyond repair. And the substance that makes the heart and other organs throw off all restraint is an excess of thyroid hormones."

Dr. James L. Goddard, former commissioner of the FDA, is another physician who warns of the dangers involved in taking *any* kind of drugs to lose weight.

"There are no drugs that can safely control the problem of weight," he says.

Then what about the men who prescribe them? How good are the diet doctors?

The second question was asked in a *Coronet* article by Peter Gall, who said, "Living off the fat of the land poses a serious matter of ethics."

It does indeed. And many of their fellow doctors have been highly critical of those ethics.

Dr. M. M. Wolfred, a pharmacologist of Beverly Hills, California, says that he knows of cases of complete nervous breakdowns attributable to heavy dosages of diet drugs, and an investigator for the AMA admitted their growing concern over the situation.

Why spend your money on appetite suppressants that endanger your health when you can substitute something that's safe and inexpensive?

The experts agree that something sweet taken shortly before meals tends to curb the appetite. Psychologist Sonja Eiteljorg says, "Diet plans fail again and again because they omit the necessary sweet crutches."

Although Miss Eiteljorg's choice of "sweet crutches" is not what I recommend, both employ the same principle. They help control the appetite, satisfy the craving for sweets, and keep the dieter from eating a hodgepodge of high-carbohydrate and highly fattening desserts.

Both are low in cost, and they contain fewer calories than the expensive "reducing" candies.

Both are part of an overall reducing program, and their primary role is that of an appetite appeaser to keep the potential delinquents from becoming diet dropouts.

The Eiteljorg diet plan is based on 30 days of reducing menus, and her "sweet crutch" is a lollypop three times a day, with the calories duly accounted for. (Dignified dieters who don't want to be caught licking a lollypop may substitute hard candies.)

If you had to choose between lollypops and reducing drugs, I'd be the first to say, "Lollypop lickers of America, unite—and fight the drug menace!"

Honey—A *Safe* Appetite Suppressant

If you want an appetite suppressant that benefits your health as it helps curb your hunger, you have a third choice.

You can choose honey.

Lollypops have no nutritional value.

Honey contains many vitamins and minerals, a few amino acids (protein), hormones, and enzymes. The *dextrose* or *levulose* in honey is the only type of sugar that is 99 percent predigested before you eat it.

Honey is the *only* concentrated sweet that I recommend using on a reducing diet.

Will it reduce you?

No, it will not. Eat too much of it and you'll gain weight.

But because of its rapid utilization, a *moderate* use of honey does not produce the body fat that other sugars do. Its *dextrose* is quickly converted in the body to *glycogen*, which supplies the body, brain and heart with ready energy.

The addition of safflower oil and vinegar to honey gives it a longer-lasting satiety value, plus the many other benefits that make formula HOV so effective.

But when the complete formula is not available, honey alone or in a cup of tea is a convenient, pleasant substitute. *Sputnik,* the English-language Russian magazine, recommends hot tea with honey and lemon as a pickup and a quick remedy for fatigue and sluggishness. Entering your bloodstream almost immediately, honey gives your blood sugar a speedy temporary boost that renews your energy and relieves your craving for food.

The boost is enough to get you past the "fat time of day" crisis without giving in to temptation. (The food element that *sustains* your blood sugar from one meal to the next will be discussed later.)

Losing your excess pounds and keeping them off are two of the best things you can do to prevent heart and artery damage and prolong your life. A world-famous heart surgeon, Dr. Michael De Bakey, says, "There is simply no question about the fact that obesity is a definite factor in heart disease, hypertension, diabetes and increased mortality."

Dr. De Bakey's diet recommendations are the same as mine, "a balanced diet ... one that includes vegetables, fruits and meats."

"Americans tend to overeat," he says. "We'd be better off eating half of what we usually eat at most meals."

Honey supplies the "sweet crutch" that satisfies your hunger and keeps you from overeating. Besides providing "food for the heart," it can help you stay on a reducing diet that might save your life.

The recorded use of honey as both food and medicine dates back more than two thousand years. It has so many nutritional and medicinal merits that it would take more than a single book to describe them all. There is only enough space in this one to tell of the help it can give, directly or indirectly, in some of the complex problems of overweight.

But perhaps the most universal reason for using honey is one that appeals to dieters and nondieters alike.

It was given centuries ago by King Solomon, who said, "My son, eat thou honey, *because it is good.*"

Fat to *Fight* Fat

Some fats can actually help you fight fat instead of putting weight on you.

But don't overlook the emphasis on *some*. It doesn't mean that you can eat any old kind of fat and slim down safely, or that I recommend a high-fat diet.

You can't, and I don't.

Whether you're trying to reduce or stay as you are, my advice is the same:

"Keep your *total* fat intake moderate, your diet *low* in animal fats, and substitute safflower or other unsaturated vegetable oil for the saturated (animal) fats whenever you can."

It's been almost twenty years since an article appeared in the *Journal of the Medical Society of Delaware* on "The Use of Fat in a Weight-Reducing Diet."

The author was Dr. Alfred W. Pennington, who said, *"The ability of tissues to oxidize fat is, in contrast to carbohydrates, unlimited."*

It's through the process of oxidation that the body burns food for energy, and some of today's high-fat, low-carbohydrate enthusiasts claim that "the body can burn an *unlimited* amount of fat."

They neglect to mention that it's unlimited only *in contrast to carbohydrates,* which most adults can burn only in rather limited amounts (it varies with the individual). Some carbohydrate is stored in the liver as *glycogen* (animal starch) for future use. What isn't burned or stored is changed into fat which settles on the least active parts of the body.

It's true that body fat is manufactured by the liver mostly from an excess of carbohydrate. But it also comes in part from an immoderate amount of fat in the diet.

Like carbohydrates, a small amount of the fat we eat is stored in the liver to be used by the nerve, brain and other cells as needed. But when excessive amounts of fat are eaten, again like carbohydrate, it's deposited as body fat on the abdomen, buttocks, hips and other underexercised parts of the body.

You get the essential fatty acids you need for normal body functioning and to sustain life in formula HOV and in the safflower oil used for salad dressing. As for animal fats, all you should have is supplied by the "hidden fats" in lean meat, poultry, fish, eggs, and low-fat cheese. If you eat "steak, fat and all, and as much butter and cream as you want," as one recent low-carbohydrate diet suggests, you will almost certainly expand your waistline—and shorten your lifeline.

As a later chapter explains, a diet high in animal fats can be dangerous.

So can the other extreme, a totally fat-free diet.

The fatty acids in unsaturated vegetable oils are essential in human nutrition, which is why they're called *essential fatty acids* (sometimes known as vitamin F). They combine with phosphorous to form a part of every cell in your body and make up part of your nerve and brain tissue.

They are essential to your health, life—and love life. One of them, linoleic acid, is necessary to form the hormones of the adrenal cortex and the sex glands. A deficiency of them recently caused one of the junior editors of a popular men's magazine to come to me for advice.

He began the conversation by saying, "I hear that you're an authority on diet and 'Sexual Vigor after Forty' " (a chapter in one of my books).

"I've researched both subjects for years," I said. "But I thought your magazine had all the answers to sex."

When he told me that he had been on a fat-free diet to lose weight in a hurry I knew what had happened to him, and why.

He was temporarily out of ardor. Before he could regain it he had to know what caused the loss, so I asked, "Have you heard of the University of Minnesota experiments that showed how rats deprived of the essential fatty acids became prematurely old, sterile, and refused to mate?"

"No," he answered, "but I know how frustrated they must have felt."

"Well, the same thing happens to humans when they are deprived of all fats in their diet, as you say you've been."

That was enough to get him back on a *balanced* reducing diet. I planned one for him that included plenty of protein (which supplied enough animal fats), low-carbohydrate fruits and vegetables, and of course, formula HOV. Its safflower oil provided the essential fatty acids he needed to help him lose weight and regain his sexual vigor at the same time.

Here are some of the ways the unsaturated fats in HOV help you fight fat, plus a few more of their vital functions.

1. Unless the body receives an adequate supply of the essential fatty acids, it changes sugar to fat much faster than it normally would.

2. Overweight persons (especially women) tend to be more or less waterlogged. Unsaturated fats, like protein, help the body rid itself of the abnormal amount of fluid retained in the tissues.

3. Without sufficient fats in the diet, the absorption of fat-soluble vitamins A, D, E, and K, and an important digestive enzyme, lipase, is inhibited.

4. Like protein, fats are more or less a self-limiting food. It's a truism that "nobody can eat just one potato chip," but fats aren't something you sit and nibble without realizing what you're doing, as you can with carbohydrates. Within varying degrees, your appetite automatically limits the amount of fat you can eat.

5. It's a physiological principle that eaten fat replaces stored body fat, loosens it, keeps this tissue moving along and prevents it from becoming stagnant and solid. (When I say "eaten fat" I'm speaking primarily of the unsaturated vegetable oils, such as the safflower oil in HOV.)

6. The normal male body is about 10 to 12 percent fat. The female body is about 25 percent. That's about the ratio of body fat necessary to support the kidneys and other vital organs and keep them from floating around in space, and to act as insulating and padding material.

Your skin requires a thin layer of fat to keep it smooth and youthful, and so do other parts of your body. If you're too skinny, you need a well-padded cushion to sit comfortably. If your weight is normal, you carry just enough of your own built-in padding. When you're too fat your upholstery is overstuffed and it's time to remodel!

7. The unsaturated vegetable oils contain lecithin, which aids in normalizing the figure that's heavy in spots, helps emulsify body fat (including that deposited in the arteries), keeps you feeling well-fed on less food, and improves your mental and physical vigor. (For larger amounts of lecithin I recommend the pleasant-tasting granules as a food supplement.)

8. Fats digest slowly and keep you feeling satisfied far

longer than carbohydrates. By slowing down the emptying
of the stomach, they keep you feeling comfortably "full,"
delay the onset of hunger and keep you from overeating.

Vinegar to *Cut* Fat

Vinegar has long been used as a health, beauty, and
reducing aid in many countries.

It was in ancient Greece that Hippocrates frequently
prescribed it for his patients, so it's no coincidence that
the secret of its medicinal, cosmetic, and slimming values
were handed down through generations of Greek mountain folk.

Recently many of its values have been publicized in England and America, notably by British researcher Cyril
Scott, Vermont's Dr. D. C. Jarvis, and screen stars Joan
Crawford and Robert Cummings, who drink it to keep
their famous figures.

At Chasen's restaurant in Hollywood and in New
York's celebrated "21," I have seen Joan Crawford sip a
jigger of vinegar (straight!) before dinner. Bob Cummings
takes two teaspoons in a glass of water with each meal,
and says, "It keeps my stomach flat and prevents a
paunch."

Bob's method is the one recommended by Dr. Jarvis,
who says it will take an inch off the waistline in a month.
"If a man has a paunch," the doctor continues, "he will
lose the paunch in two years' time. The cider vinegar will
have made it possible to burn fat in the body instead of
storing it, increasing the body weight."

Cyril Scott gives in great detail the functions of cider
vinegar, but the ones most relevant to our subject are these:

"It promotes digestion," he says, "for the reason that
cider vinegar bears a closer resemblance to the digestive
juices than does any other fluid; it favors oxidation of the
blood; it regulates calcium metabolism; *it retards the onset
of old age; it cures and prevents obesity. . . .*"

Mr. Scott stressed the fact that "ordinary vinegar must
not be used, as it does not contain the properties of vinegar made from apples. . . ."

And be sure it's naturally fermented (available in some
markets and in all health food stores) and not the distilled
varieties, which have the living bacteria destroyed.

As long ago as 1839, a German chemist, Baron Justus von Liebig, demonstrated the value of the natural ferments in undistilled vinegar, based on the chemical action of the fermentation processes: *that a small quantity of one substance can bring about changes in large quantities of other substances.*

So it is that a relatively small quantity of naturally fermented cider vinegar (as used in formula HOV) can attack, and in combination with the oil, disperse larger quantities of accumulated fat. The decomposition (or destruction) of fat is caused by the same chemical process that tenderizes meat soaked in vinegar, or marinated in oil and vinegar, which today's housewives prefer.

Vinegar's most active factor is acetic acid. Industrially, in its pure form, acetic acid is used as a solvent. As a solvent of fatty substances, it acts as an emulsifying agent of the fat it attacks. In the *Journal of Pharmaceutical Chemistry,* Professor Meillère has shown that vinegar contains *inositol,* which we know is a lipotropic agent or fat disperser.

The solvent effects of vinegar are mentioned in the Old Testament, and Pliny, an early Roman naturalist and author, told how Cleopatra won a wager by dissolving pearls in vinegar.

The incident isn't as incredible as it sounds if you remember that pearls are merely lipidlike (fatty) tumescent exudations that have solidified, layer by layer. And if vinegar can dissolve the solidified fatty layers of a pearl, think how much easier it should be to "melt away" the softer layers of human fat and flab!

In one of my books I named sugar, white flour, and hard fats the Terrible Trio mainly responsible for overweight.

Now in formula HOV we have another trio that *fights* obesity, a trio so *safe, economical* and *effective* that I think it, too, should be known by the initials of the words describing it.

HOV, the *SEE* Trio.

And what you'll *SEE* is the beginning of your new image as your stomach starts to flatten, your hips slim down, and your weight returns to normal . . .

S afely
E conomically
E ffectively

6

Eat All You Want—
of Some *Foods*

"In dieting, every second counts," said humorist Jack Herbert.

And except for *some* foods it does.

Dr. Frederick Stare, who lives by Yankee discipline and a rule of "eat less, stay slim, live longer," takes a grim view of second helpings and their long-range results. "It's not a mark of hospitality to insist on guests having seconds," he says sternly. "Make the offer once and shut up!"

If you're a fatty who is tempted by "just one more hot roll and butter" or a second helping of pasta or dessert, you became a diet delinquent when you ate the *first* helping.

I know it's hard to resist if you've been conditioned to rich food and extra helpings since childhood. But by substituting eat-all-you-want foods for high-carbohydrates —and with HOV to control your appetite—it can be done.

First, take HOV. And I hope you *are* taking it. Not just now and then, whenever you happen to think of it, but three times a day. Regularly, and as specified, if you expect to get results. Yet how many times do you say to yourself, "It won't matter if I skip it this once," or forget it completely?

When that happens you do need an extra helping—of *willpower,* not food. If you have enough willpower or know where to get some in a hurry, it can see you through a temporary hunger crisis.

When willpower is lacking, a *strong motivation,* stronger than your desire for food, will keep you from overeating. But the two are so closely related that when one is missing the other weakens and loses much of its drive.

That leaves one powerful alternative. *Fear*.

How did a negative emotion such as fear get in the same league with positive ones? Because I have seen the fear of disabling illness or premature death give many obese persons the *motivation* to lose weight and the *willpower* to stay on a diet when nothing else would.

A few months ago a man who was afraid came to see me. His name, he told me, was Jess Gorman, and he was worried about his wife. "She's gained more than sixty pounds in the past four years," he said. "Now she gets short of breath just bending over to put on her shoes, and it's an effort for her to walk from the house to the car. I can't get her to go to a doctor, but she's agreed to see you."

After making an appointment for her, he said, "She'll tell you that she doesn't eat much, and she doesn't—at the table. But she raids the refrigerator between meals and at midnight for second and third helpings—especially of dessert. Can you help her?"

"I can," I said, "but only by gaining her cooperation. I won't know how to do that until I talk to her. Any suggestions?"

"Only one," he said. "Put the fear of God in her!"

The "fear of God" is outside my jurisdiction.

But the fear of overweight is in my domain, and I have no hands-off policy concerning it. It's something that *should* be feared, and I'll tell the dangers of obesity to every fatty who'll listen—and to some who won't.

Mrs. Gorman promised to substitute foods from the Eat-All-You-Want list (pages 191-2) for her between-meal snacks, to stay on the diet I gave her, and to take HOV as directed.

Since she did her heaviest eating between meals, I changed the usual method of taking HOV to one that met her unusual requirements. "Take it when you feel a refrigerator raid coming on," I told her, "morning, afternoon, or midnight. Put a jar on your bedside table at night in case you wake up hungry."

Less than two weeks later her husband came to see me again. "She hasn't done any of the things you told her to," he said, "and she's gained five more pounds. Worse than that, she's been having what she calls 'indigestion.' I'm afraid it's her heart, but she won't listen to me."

I handed him a paper from my desk and asked, "Do you think she'd listen to this?"

It was a reprint of a black-bordered page with a funeral wreath at the top, and the alarming statistics it contained were compiled by the Metropolitan Life Insurance Company:

DEATH RATE GOES UP WITH EACH EXCESS POUND

Among moderately fat men, the death rate is . . . .
   42% HIGHER than among men of normal weight.
Among very fat men, the death rate is . . . .
   79% HIGHER than among men of normal weight.
Among moderately fat women, the death rate is . . . .
   42% HIGHER than among women of normal weight.
Among very fat women, the death rate is . . . .
   61% HIGHER than among women of normal weight.

When he finished reading it, I asked, "Why don't you keep that copy and paste it on the refrigerator door— along with the fattest picture of her you can find?"

"It just might do it." A smile began playing hide-'n-seek with the worried lines in his face, and he repeated what seemed to be one of his favorite phrases, "It just might put the fear of God in her and make her follow your advice."

He was right. It took fear to give Mrs. Gorman the strong motivation she needed to get started and to give her willpower its initial boost. After that, HOV and the following low-carbohydrate foods and unlimited beverages satisfied her appetite, kept her from overeating and on a balanced reducing diet for the seven months it took her to lose sixty pounds.

Eat All You Want—of *These* Foods

Group I.

Vegetables, Raw or Cooked

artichokes, globe and
   Jerusalem
asparagus
bamboo shoots

green and red pepper
kale
lettuce

beans, green and wax
bean sprouts
beet greens
broccoli
cabbage
cauliflower
celery
chard

chicory
Chinese cabbage
Chinese water chestnuts
cucumber
endive
escarole

mushrooms
mustard greens
parsley
pickles
pimientos
radishes
romaine
sauerkraut, low salt, naturally
    fermented
spinach
summer squash
tampala
turnip greens
watercress
zucchini

For slimming snacks to stave off hunger, keep your refrigerator stocked with eat-all-you-want vegetables and prepare a day's supply at a time. Wash and dry them in a clean tea towel, save some for cooking or for dinner salads if you like, cut the rest into bite-sized pieces and refrigerate them in a bowl covered with plastic wrap. They'll stay crisp, fresh and ready for nibbling whenever you are.

My own favorite combination is an offbeat assortment of raw mushrooms, radishes, bean sprouts, cauliflower knobs and zucchini sticks spiked with a sprinkle of garlic powder. I can eat them at my desk with one hand while I write with the other, so for me they are both time- and hunger-savers.

Let Yourself Go with Seasonings

Group II.

Herbs, Spices, Seeds, and Sauces

You may use any of these as freely as your taste dictates:

Vinegar, lemon juice, horseradish, mustard, soy, and Worcestershire sauce.

Caraway, celery, dill, poppy and sesame seeds.

All herbs, fresh and dried.

Almost all spices, including curry, paprika, and freshly ground black pepper.

Now let's see what we can do with them to enhance the flavor of some of the vegetables on our list.

Who says you need butter, cream sauce or Hollandaise on vegetables? The mild flavor of *asparagus* goes Oriental with a few drops of soy sauce mixed with lemon juice and topped with poppy or sesame seeds.

Tired of plain *broccoli*? Fancy it up with a tiny fleck of curry (careful, it's strong stuff!), tarragon, or marjoram, and a pinch of poppy seeds.

A little curry and lemon juice are good with *cabbage*, too. Or try it with a sauce of cider vinegar, snipped chives and caraway, dill or celery seeds.

Season *green beans* with fresh dill, rosemary, savory, or snipped mint. Or for an unusual flavor, add a whisper of nutmeg.

Vinegar and a drop or two of Worcestershire add a zippy flavor to chard, spinach, mustard, turnip, beet or dandelion greens. Or blend a smidgin of horseradish or mustard with vinegar and pour over them.

A snippet of fresh dill, basil or oregano and a dash of soy sauce perk up the flavor of summer squash.

Soy sauce peps up the taste of zucchini, too, but this time try it with marjoram.

Cut down on salt, but don't cut it out completely. Avoid such highly salted foods as ham, pastrami, luncheon meats, smoked or cured fish, and smoked tongue. Just remember that salt retains up to 70 times its weight in water, and a lot of excess fluid held in your tissues can make you waterlogged and pudgy.

Drink All You Want of These

Group III.

Unlimited Beverages

Assorted teas, including American, English, Irish, Russian, Japanese, Chinese, and herb teas, hot or iced.

"Take tea for comfort," advises Dr. Theodore Isaac Rubin, better known as the Formerly Fat Psychiatrist. "Fat people are most receptive to comfort."

From his own experience in dieting Dr. Rubin learned, as I did, the value of having a stock of easily prepared snacks and beverages that "comfort" the stomach and prevent overeating.

You can go international with a variety of teas and flavors. A tiny fleck of nutmeg adds interest to Chinese and Japanese tea, and a light dusting of cinnamon is good with most of the others. Or if you can get it, stirring them with a swizzle stick of cinnamon bark enhances the taste and smell. Add crushed fresh mint leaves and a lemon twist for a mint julep-y flavor, garnish with slices of lemon or orange stuck with cloves, or add one or two fresh strawberries.

In England and Ireland, where tea is the national drink, it's served with milk instead of cream. If you prefer it that way, have a little skim milk in yours, but no cream or sugar. And if you don't like any kind of tea, take your choice of the other unlimited beverages.

Coffee and *coffee substitutes. No sugar in these or any of the unlimited beverages, or they won't be unlimited.* A drop or two of pure vanilla extract (or if you can get it, a vanilla bean) adds a little sweetness and a distinctive flavor, and is especially good in iced coffee. If you can't drink it black, a dash of skim milk is all right.

Clam juice, hot or chilled. It's still within limits if you mix it with a 1-ounce jigger of tomato juice.

Club soda or *seltzer,* with a lemon twist or a spoonful of lemon or lime juice, if desired.

Lemon and *lime drinks.* Serve them in a tall glass over crushed ice, diluted with plenty of water. Add a crushed sprig of fresh mint and a fresh berry or two, and they'll be so refreshing you won't need a sweetener.

Consommé and *bouillon* made from cubes, concentrated *vegetable broth* in cubes or powder, and other nonfat clear soups. Have them hot, jellied, or on the rocks. Make a tomato bouillon by adding ¼ cup of tomato juice to ¾ cup of bouillon made with a cube, seasoned to taste with herbs. (I like it simmered with a tiny pinch of oregano or a small piece of bay leaf, and a sprinkle of kelp and concentrated vegetable powder.)

Another of my favorites, satisfying but still within limits, is made by adding a teaspoon each of chopped mushrooms, celery and slivers of chicken to a cup of consommé or any of the unlimited clear soups.

Dr. Clarence Cohn, director of the Division of Nutritional Sciences at Michael Reese Hospital in Chicago, has been a confirmed snacker most of his adult life. He recently conducted an experiment that proved the merits of snacking, and revealed an unexpected fringe benefit.

Two test groups were given the same amount of food, 2,000 calories a day. One group was composed of "typical eaters" who ate all of their food in the conventional three meals a day. The other group was made up of snackers who divided their food allowance into three relatively small meals and three snacks a day.

Both groups were given a physical examination and psychological tests before the experiment began and after it was over. The final results were amazing, especially in one area. Not only had the snackers reduced their waistlines between one and two inches, but their general condition was better, their morale and spirits were higher and they had become noticeably "happier" than the group who ate three average meals a day.

So snack to avoid the frustrations of reducing, to feel better, lose weight faster and stay happier!

Eat and drink all you want of the foods and beverages on the unlimited lists. And there is another snack you may have in moderation. It's the most important food element in your diet, whether you're trying to lose weight or not.

Protein to *Burn* Fat

Protein was not included in the eat-all-you-want lists. Although it's pretty much a self-limiting food, as I mentioned earlier, it isn't quite unlimited. It's the basis of any sound diet, and the only safe way to reduce. If we were counting calories I'd have to say that protein contains a fair share of them, but instead of counting them you *subtract*. In many cases it costs more calories to digest protein than it contains.

As your metabolism is stepped up, you can burn up to 130 or more protein calories for each 113 you eat. They are *working* calories that carry their own weight instead of piling it up on you.

More than any other food, protein has this special slimming factor. It's called *specific dynamic action*.

You remember what it is, don't you?

It's an element that causes the greatest rise in metabolism, keeps it in high gear longer, and burns up fat deposits faster than anything else.

Stored body fat is *reserve* fuel.

Ready fuels are sugar, starch, and alcohol (yes, alcohol, too, no matter what *The Drinking Man's Diet* claims).

High-carbohydrates function as a *ready* but low-grade fuel, and like other low-grade fuels, they can clog up the works by sparing fats that should be kept on the move.

You've heard the expression "fat and lazy," and that's what fat is when it's spared by carbohydrates and deposited as spare tires around the body. It gets itself on the "most dangerous" docket, too, by settling in the tissues and arteries. Wherever it settles, it just sits there and refuses to budge as long as the ready fuels of sugar and starch are available.

But take them away and the stored fat has to stop loafing and get back to work.

Cut out all carbohydrates except those on the allowed list, make protein the mainstay of your diet, drink a *minimum* of liquor (sorry about that!), and watch the results.

The blobs of stored fat come out of reserve and start burning for energy (safflower oil helps keep it from settling in the arteries) and you start losing weight. Steadily, in pounds and inches. In fatty tissue and excess water content, but not in vital tissue. No matter how overweight you are, you can't afford to lose at the expense of vital tissue, and protein protects it.

Protein, as you know, is the only food that renews and rebuilds the tissues and cells. And when you stop and think of the number of cells that might need repairing it's enough to stagger the mind. The adult body is composed of over *one hundred trillion cells*.

Every hour our bodies supply and dispose of a billion or so cells, so if you can divide a hundred trillion by a billion maybe you can figure out how much protein it takes to keep the supply ahead of the disposal.

I haven't quite figured it out yet, but I'm not taking any chances. I make it a point to eat protein at every meal, and sometimes between meals, which brings us back to the subject of snacking.

The metabolic heat that helps burn body fat is provided by protein's specific dynamic action. When you skip a meal, or go for long periods without eating protein, that metabolic heat is reduced—and you aren't.

In experiments at the University of Wisconsin hospital in Madison, Doctors Edgar Gordon and E. Marshall Goldberg found that in cases of low or abnormal metabolism, the *spacing* or timing of meals on a reducing diet is as important as their *quantity*.

One of their test cases was a middle-aged woman weighing 278 pounds. For several weeks she had been on a diet of 950 calories a day without losing an ounce. Her breakfast consisted of fruit juice and coffee, luncheon was black coffee, and the only protein she ate was at dinner, her one meal of the day.

The doctors took her off the starvation diet, put her on one of 1,200 calories that was high in protein, moderate in fats, and extremely low in carbohydrates. They told her to eat it in small snacks, six or more times a day, and from then on she began to lose weight steadily.

According to Dr. Gordon, the system of some persons "prefers not to burn its carbohydrates straight, but first to turn them into fat."

The best way to change that "preference" is to see that each meal contains one or more of the complete proteins and a minimum of carbohydrates. Don't fall into the trap of eating all or most of your protein at night, as the majority do. To step up your metabolism, provide better utilization and lose weight faster, why not divide your meals into several smaller snacks?

It's his scientific knowledge, not the fact that he's a snacker himself, that prompts Dr. Cohn to say, "The more one spreads out the protein, the better it's utilized."

The Cohn family starts the day with protein, and the children "may eat some leftover roast beef; their morning meal often resembles a small dinner."

When Mrs. Cohn is home during the day her eating pattern seldom varies from this:

Breakfast: Fresh fruit, coffee with skim milk, and cheese.

Around 10:30: Another piece of cheese or a cold cut.

Noon: A slice of meat, chicken or cheese.

2:00 P.M. If hungry, she has half a slice of bread with meat or cheese, and maybe a tomato.

4:30 p.m. A piece of fresh fruit.

Dinner with the family: Usually meat, fish or chicken,

vegetables, and a salad. If fruit or other dessert is served it's eaten later as a special snack.

Bedtime: Another nibble of cold meat or cheese.

This is just an example of one way to keep your protein intake high throughout the day. There are other ways more convenient for the person who works.

If you carry your lunch I hope you include some raw, unlimited vegetables. Save a few of them and a piece of meat instead of a sandwich for an afternoon snack—and don't forget to throw most of the bread away. For a restaurant coffee break, have a wedge of cheese and black coffee or tea, or a protein pickup of skim milk or buttermilk. A small scoop of cottage cheese is fine (remember it's a snack, not a meal!), and so is half a container of yogurt.

The idea is to eat *part* of what you would have at a regular meal, not an additional meal that you call a snack.

On a high-protein diet you can burn fat instead of depositing it on your body and still eat all you want of the unlimited foods. And *almost* all the protein you can hold— but not quite.

At least not until your appestat is back to normal and you start slimming down. Then a new life can begin for you. As a distinguished doctor says of a high-protein diet, "The rewards are great."

Here, condensed, is how Dr. Max Konigsberg describes them:

"A high-protein diet will help you to the spirited health that persists into old age . . . vitality, a zest for life in a well-functioning and handsome body . . . effective resistance to infection and disease. . . . It assures a prognosis of blessed longevity."

Protein does all of this and a great deal more by supplying your body with the raw materials it must have to produce its red and white corpuscles, to provide disease-fighting antibodies, and to preserve and renew your cells and tissues.

"It makes possible daily well-being and working efficiency," Dr. Konigsberg continues. "Whether you are young or aging . . . sick and want to recover your strength, normal and hoping to stay that way—*or overweight and have to lose poundage healthily, protein is your dish.*"

Why not try it and see?

7

Debunking Four Popular Diets

Diets that have been weighed and found wanting have become almost as inevitably a part of our lives as death and taxes.

And the comparison isn't as far-fetched as it seems. Any severely restricted or unbalanced diet taxes your health, and when carried to excess some of them have been known to result in death.

It is hoped you won't stay on such a diet very long. But before you have time to recover from it, a new one appears—or an old one reappears under a different name and with a new gimmick.

Whether a diet is old or new, original or a rehashed version in disguise and with or without gimmicks doesn't matter very much.

What does matter is whether or not it will reduce you *safely.* If it can't, gimmicks and ballyhoo won't help. They can make a diet popular, but they can't make it effective. They provide publicity, not safety. Unfortunately, many dieters are so willing to believe any new get-slim scheme that they fail to ask, "Is it safe?"

Let's take a look at some of the popular versions of an old diet and see how they measure up.

It was in 1890 that the English medical journal, *Lancet,* published an article called "A Diet of Lean Meat and Water."

Does that sound familiar to you? It should.

Variations of it have been the basis of a dozen modern diets, including such favorites as *The Mayo Clinic Diet, The Air Force Diet* (which were disowned by the Mayo Clinic and the Air Force), *The Drinking Man's Diet,*

Martinis and Whipped Cream, and the all-protein diet of
The Doctor's Quick Weight Loss group.

The Doctor's Quick Weight Loss stuck with the original lean meat and no-carbohydrate principle and stayed
on the water wagon and the soda fountain (with artificially sweetened carbonated drinks). The others took liquor
off the no-no list, added fat meat to the lean, and allowed
up to 60 grams of carbohydrate a day.

Since several of the currently popular diets follow the
same general pattern, for convenience let's break them
down into these categories:

1. The Hard-Liquor and High-Fat Diet.
2. The All-Protein Diet.
3. The No-Protein or All-Carbohydrate Diet.
4. The Macrobiotics Diet.

Can you lose weight on these diets?

If so, will it be permanent?

And how great is the risk?

These are the key questions. The first two can be
answered with a simple "yes" and "no."

Yes, the chances are that you can lose some weight on
them. No, it will not be permanent. They are not diets
that you can stay on for the rest of your life—if you could
live that long on them! And when you go back to your old
eating pattern you'll start gaining again.

What about the risk?

It varies from person to person, from diet to diet, and
with the length of time you stay on it. For some persons
the damage is temporary and easily remedied. For others
it can be lasting and serious. How would *you* be affected?
Maybe you'll find out as we examine each category of
diets separately, weigh their good and bad points and see
where they are found wanting.

The Hard-Liquor and High-Fat Diet

We'll start with a category that has a universal appeal
to the drinking man (or woman). Under this heading are
four of the five diets previously mentioned. The collective
title of *Hard-Liquor and High-Fat* sounds less persuasive
than their original names, but essentially that's what they
are. They're better known as *The Drinking Man's Diet*
(there's a *Drinking Girl's Diet,* too), a new version of the

Mayo Clinic Diet, *Martinis and Whipped Cream, The Air Force Diet,* or as one of several similar diets classed ambiguously as *High-Protein* or *Low-Carbohydrate.*

I say ambiguously because the big selling point that attracts anyone who drinks is not so much how to *eat* and get thin, but how to *drink* and reduce.

Dieters have been warned for years that liquor is high in calories. It still is. Alcohol may evaporate, but calories don't.

Our best scientific minds have been busy with spatial projects, and producing a no-cal liquor isn't on their priority list. And so far it's impossible to filter the calories out, skim them off, or let them settle in the bottom of the glass and sip around them. So what do you do with them?

If you're a drinker you drink them.

Yes, I know. I said that with HOV you wouldn't have to count the calories you ate, and you don't. But I didn't say it about the ones you *drink.*

Liquor contains no nutrients. No protein, vitamins or minerals. Nutritionally, its calories are zero. Numerically, they add up to a hefty count. You simply can't afford many of them when you're trying to reduce and need to make every calorie count in terms of food value, not avoirdupois.

The authors of *Martinis and Whipped Cream* are speaking of carbohydrate calories when they say, "Only beer drinkers will have to count, and only cordial and liqueur drinkers will have to switch. For the cocktail hour or two, sip away to your heart's content on Manhattans, dry Martinis or Bacardis."

Beer, cordials, liqueurs and sweet wines are not allowed because they are high in carbohydrate. (How did Bacardis get in when they're made with sugar and grenadine?)

The ones you are told you may drink "to your heart's content" are bourbon, Scotch, rum, vodka, gin and some brandies.

They claim that "there is not a trace of fattening carbohydrates" in hard liquor, but all the diets in this category overlook one significant fact:

Much of the alcohol is oxidized through the carbohydrate metabolic pathway.

Alcohol is, as you already know, a *ready* fuel, the same as carbohydrate. And they have other similarities. Both of them generate heat, provide a form of quick energy, and unless restricted, both can easily put weight on you.

Your metabolism may permit you to use both *in moderation* and still reduce, or it may not. In either case, you will slim down faster by going on the wagon as you limit your carbohydrate intake.

An excess of both will almost certainly layer you with fat, keep you from losing it—and may present other embarrassing problems.

Let television personality Lenny Weinrib tell what happened to him.

"There isn't a diet in the world I haven't tried," said Lenny, naming most of those on our debunking list. "The Mayo Clinic Diet. The Air Force Diet. The High-Carbohydrate Diet. The Low-Carbohydrate Diet. The Drinking Man's Diet ... I didn't get thin, but I crashed into my garage door."

"If you drink a large amount of alcohol and eat a large amount of fat," says Dr. Jean Mayer, "what will happen is that you will be fat and inebriated."

Dr. Harry J. Johnson, author of *Eat, Drink, Be Merry & Live Longer,* calls it "just another in the procession of fad diets that promise a painless, quick way to lose weight." He cautions that it will deprive your body of nutrients that are necessary to your health, and continues with this stern warning:

". . . To condone the excessive consumption of alcoholic beverages indicated in sample menus of this diet is courting serious trouble. You may wind up becoming an alcoholic."

Mrs. Elmer Wheeler, wife of the famous "Fat Boy," kept a watchful eye on her husband when he started his Drinking Man's Binge.

"What I liked best," said Elmer, "was the fact that no one had discovered a carbohydrate in whiskey."

But it didn't solve his weight problem, so he decided to quit when his wife began to tell their friends, "Now Elmer has *two* problems!"

Teetotalers will probably blast me for not giving a blow-by-blow account of the problems caused by alcohol, but I have already done so in another book (*How to Keep Your Youthful Vitality After Forty*). The points I want to emphasize here are these:

1. Cutting any of the essential nutrients out of your diet

to allow for an excessive indulgence in alcohol will endanger your health.

2. Alcohol may not contain carbohydrates, but it *can* make you fat, and it *will* inhibit weight loss. If you're an "easy fattener" don't expect to drink up and slim down at the same time. Wait until your weight is normal, then try a glass of dry wine with dinner, or if you must, an occasional highball made with water or club soda. But don't ever again believe that you can drink all the hard liquor you want and not gain weight. Not unless your appetite for liquor is extremely moderate. And even then you'd be better off switching to dry wine.

With the exception of vodka, which has almost none, all hard liquors contain congeners (fusel oils, acetic acid, etc.). The amount varies with the type of liquor and the distilling method used, but as a general rule, the higher the proof of the alcohol the more congeners it contains (and the more calories, too!).

Some of these congeners can cause allergic reactions, many are partly toxic, and the victim of a hangover can blame them for contributing heavily to his misery.

Which is more harmful, an excessive amount of hard liquor or hard fats in the diet?

It's a difficult question to answer without first asking "To whom?" and "Under what circumstances?"

The tolerance to both varies with the individual, his age, physical activity, and mode of life.

The one can cause cirrhosis of the liver, and the other may result in a fatty infiltration that impairs the liver's function. By destroying brain cells, the immoderate use of alcohol can cause a loss of mental acuity, and in advanced cases, premature senility. Excessive amounts of fat in the diet can produce the same condition by clogging the arteries to the brain with cholesterol deposits.

Let Dr. William D. Snively, author of *Sea of Life*, tell what happened to his cholesterol count when he went on one of the diets in this category.

"Believing it too good to be true," said Dr. Snively, "I, nevertheless, tried the Air Force diet. Like so many others, I gained weight, while my cholesterol, usually about 180 milligrams per 100 milliliters of plasma, *rose to a thumping 375.*"

And is there anyone who doesn't know by now the correlation between high cholesterol and heart attacks, or that a coronary occurs when the main artery to the heart is blocked?

The increase in coronary and other fat-related diseases have in the past seventeen years dropped the American male from eleventh place in a life-expectancy rate to thirty-seventh place today.

Most of the authors of these diets do mention the relation of hard fats to cholesterol, but not strongly enough to discourage potential buyers of their books.

They protect themselves by saying, "Have a medical checkup before starting the diet," but it doesn't protect the dieter. Few of them ever follow such advice.

My advice is what it has always been:

To slim down safely and faster, restrict your liquor intake and keep your diet low in animal fats by substituting unsaturated vegetable oils for them whenever possible.

The All-Protein Diet

Every book I have written has emphasized the value of a high-protein diet, and if this diet were judged solely by the quality of its protein content it wouldn't be on a debunking list.

Here are the foods permitted on it:

1. *Lean meats,* broiled, baked or roasted.

2. *Chicken and turkey,* with the skin removed, broiled, roasted or baked.

3. *Lean fish and seafood,* broiled, baked or poached.

4. *Eggs,* preferably hardboiled (for their satiety value), but may be cooked any way not using fats.

5. *Cottage cheese* and other low-fat or skim-milk cheeses such as farmer or pot cheese.

So far, fine. It's exactly what I recommend as the basis of sound nutrition and safe reducing. EXCEPT . . .

This isn't merely the *basis* of a diet. They are the only foods allowed. As a long-ago song used to say, "That's all there is, there ain't no more." And for long-term dieting it just isn't enough.

You're allowed common seasonings and all you want of the usual calorie-free beverages—club soda, Vichy water, and coffee and tea without cream or sugar.

And although long before cyclamates were removed

from the market the public had been warned to restrict their use of artificially sweetened drinks, the authors of this version of the all-protein diet suggests them as "a treat you may enjoy just about as many times a day as you wish." One of the co-writers, a doctor, advised his patients to drink ten or twelve of them a day, in a variety of flavors, to curb hunger and a craving for sweets!

In addition to other liquids, eight glasses of water a day are stressed as an absolute essential to wash waste products of "ashes of burnt fat" out of the system and to relieve any "unpleasant dryness and taste in the mouth."

According to the authors, the addition of any food or drink not on the list will prevent the full and efficient functioning of what they call *"the high-protein internal reducing process which burns up fat."*

We know it's a fact that the specific dynamic action of protein causes the rapid burning of fat. It's also one of the reasons the *all-protein* diet is not advisable for long-term reducing programs.

Using myself as a hypothetical guinea pig, I asked a doctor, a scientist, and a food chemist this question:

"What would happen if I ate absolutely nothing but protein indefinitely?"

The answer was unanimous, "My God, you'd literally burn yourself up!"

Excess stored fat is all you want to burn, not vital tissue. Not the *élément constant,* the fat incorporated into the cellular structures of the heart, brain, liver and other organs in complex molecules. For their proper functioning, the vital organs require some carbohydrate (in the form of glucose). Not a *lot,* but *some,* part of which the liver converts to glycogen and stores for later use.

What happens on a diet that omits all carbohydrates? When there are no vegetables or fruits to be changed into glucose for the body's immediate demands or stored as glycogen to be reconverted by the liver for future needs?

Within a few days the glycogen stored in the liver and muscles will be almost depleted. Almost, but not quite.

With incredible efficiency, the liver will continue to produce some from whatever source is available. Enough sugar (glucose) must always circulate to maintain a blood level circulation of 80-120 mg per 100 cc. With no carbohydrates to supply this amount, the liver converts protein to glucose to make up the deficit. The result is a continuous loss of body protein and some tissue break-down.

During a recent lecture I gave a brief summary of this part of the book and was surprised afterwards to see how an audience (or a reader?) can take a few remarks out of context and somehow misconstrue the meaning of a statement.

"You used to be *for* protein and *against* carbohydrate," a woman told me, "and now you've changed and are for carbohydrates and against protein, aren't you?"

How could anyone possibly get that idea?

I haven't changed, unless constantly investigating new food values and evaluating old ones can be called changing.

I always have been and still am "for" protein, and I've never been "against" carbohydrates, except for the processed and highly refined products made with white flour and sugar.

Anyone familiar with my work should certainly know that I recommend a diet high in protein—*but one which doesn't omit the other essential nutrients.*

If you've read many diet books you must have heard of *ketosis.* It's a severe form of acidosis that results from a diet that cuts carbohydrates below a safe level.

Without carbohydrates, fats can't be completely broken down in the body. As a result of incomplete fat oxidation, chemical products of metabolism called *ketone bodies* accumulate in the blood in excessive amounts. This causes the blood (*not* the stomach!) to become too acid. Diabetics on a severely restricted diet are familiar with ketosis as a condition that can trigger the dreaded diabetic coma.

In a mild form, ketosis can cause fatigue, dizziness, nausea, nervousness, headache, and the "unpleasant dryness and taste in the mouth" already mentioned.

At its worst it can produce a toxic condition and rob the body of so much potassium that the victim may lose consciousness, and unless the symptoms are reversed, death may follow.

The National Research Council recommends 400 calories of carbohydrates a day. Many experts believe that you can temporarily cut down to around 250 calories (about 60 grams) with no harmful effects, but all agree on the danger of cutting them out entirely.

Let protein be the *basis* of your diet, but not all of it.

Supplement it with low-carbohydrate vegetables and fruits for their rich vitamin and mineral content. Eat some of them raw for extra benefits from the enzymes, or catalysts, which help speed up the conversion of food to energy.

In his book, *How to Keep Fit and Enjoy It,* Dr. Warren Guild draws the following equation to illustrate the process:

$$\text{Food} \xrightarrow[\text{(Slowly)}]{\text{No Enzymes}} \text{Heat (Energy)}$$

"If the proper enzymes, or catalysts, are added," says Dr. Guild, "this process can be accelerated manifold ... using up the food and producing energy. This appears as":

$$\text{Food} \xrightarrow[\text{(Rapidly)}]{\text{Enzymes}} \text{Heat (Energy)}$$

With their speed-up system of using up food and producing energy, enzyme-rich raw vegetables and fruits can help you lose weight as they protect your health. (Choose the vegetables from the Eat-All-You-Want list on pages 191-2, and limit the fruits to two or three a day until your weight is normal.)

The surest way to keep from burning up vital tissue, prevent tissue breakdown, avoid ketosis and reduce *safely* is to cut *down,* but not *out.*

Yet the dangerous lopsided diets continue to flourish, as you'll see by the next category.

The No-Protein or All-Carbohydrate Diet

In a complete turn-around, the authors of the preceding diet give us another run-around.

Consistency? They never heard of it!

From an All-Protein quick-weight-loss program that made carbohydrates the villain, they switch to another quickie which they claim will reduce you in inches.

And guess who's the bad guy now? Protein!

Remember the only foods that were allowed on the All-Protein Diet? Here they are again—on the *forbidden* list this time.

"NOT PERMITTED"

Meats	All poultry
Fish	Eggs
Seafood	Cheeses

And to make sure that a decent gram of protein doesn't sneak in, they've forbidden the following vegetable proteins:

Avocados	Gelatine
Beans (except green or wax)	Lentils
Peas	Nuts
Coconut	

Milk isn't on the list, but it was forbidden on another page where the dieter was told to use cream, preferably mixed with water, on cereals. (Both hot and cold cereals are allowed, except for those marked "contains protein.")

On the "Not Permitted" list are all of the complete animal proteins and some incomplete but better-than-average vegetable proteins.

The authors insist that their current brainstorm is a "low-protein, not a no-protein diet," but with the above foods omitted from it I consider it a gross exaggeration to call it anything except a No-Protein or an All-Carbohydrate diet.

On the "Permitted" list is practically everything that doesn't contain protein: vegetables, fruits, soups (except those made with meat, chicken, fish or other protein), bread, muffins, toast, crackers, biscuits, jams, jellies, marmalades, preserves, rice, spaghetti, puddings, sherbet, and a variety of "bland cookies, but not any marked 'contains protein.' "

All of this on a reducing diet?

Yes, but the authors have conveniently left themselves a loophole. Sprinkled through the text are frequent warnings to eat *very small portions,* or to *use very sparingly.* In one place they come right out and admit that you will "fail to lose pounds and inches if you use these foods liberally."

By eating only the permitted foods (and don't forget the small portions!), they say you will get the "allowed 15 to 20 grams of protein" a day.

Although admitting that this diet is very low in protein, their contention is that it contains "far more than enough" to maintain and promote excellent health and vigor. Even worse is their irresponsible statement that if you have no special medical problem you can stay on this semi-starvation diet "year after year with no harmful effects."

If you're thinking of trying it, wait until you take a look at the facts.

First, the 15 to 20 grams of protein a day allowed on the diet is totally inadequate, both in quantity and quality, for man, woman, or child.

The average person in good health needs a daily minimum of 65 to 75 grams of *complete animal protein*. For optimum health and vitality I like to keep my own intake around 100 grams a day. The sick person, the marginal cases, those who are out of nitrogen balance and the ones with poor absorption may require 125 to 150 grams a day.

Second, the "allowed proteins" are of vegetable origin, incomplete and of inferior quality. With a few exceptions—which aren't permitted on this diet!—vegetable proteins lack some of the essential amino acids and are incapable of promoting health or supporting life.

Dr. Philip L. White, Secretary of the AMA's Council on Foods and Nutrition, did a little debunking of his own when he emphatically denied the authors' claim that the body doesn't need much protein and that their diet provides "sufficient for health and vigor."

"This is simply not so," said Dr. White in a recent issue of *Today's Health*. "The body is unable to get along on 15 to 20 grams of dietary protein, particularly when it is of vegetable origin."

Dr. White accused the authors of running the gamut from high-protein to almost none, and noting that in their first book "carbohydrate is damned, now it is praised," he asks, "What is left?"

Calling the diet plan *induced malnutrition*, Dr. White continues:

"There is every reason to be concerned about the safety of the *Inches-Off* diet, which would cause considerable protein loss from the body. *The protein of vital organs could be dangerously depleted. . . . Such losses could be quite devastating. . . .*" (My italics.)

On a diet deficient in protein you will age faster. Sags and wrinkles will appear prematurely and muscles will sag and begin to waste away. Vitality will give way to fatigue and depression. You will look, feel, and act much older than you are.

Whether malnutrition and a protein deficiency are induced by a deliberately restricted diet or from whatever cause, the results are disastrous to health, youth, and longevity.

And the diet that follows is even more severely restricted than those in the first three categories.

The Macrobiotics Diet

Macrobiotics is a system of diet based on a 4,000-year-old Oriental principle of balance.

How can I, a strong believer in a balanced diet, argue with that?

Because the most dedicated followers of Macrobiotics are convinced that perfect health of mind and body and harmony between the human spirit and nature can be attained by subsisting for an indefinite length of time on a single food.

With respect for the philosophy behind it, but not for the system, I disagree.

It was developed by a Japanese, Dr. Sagen Isiduke, more than 70 years ago. His successor, Dr. Georges Ohsawa, has written several books on the subject and expanded it to include his own ideas.

The diet itself is based philosophically on the ancient Oriental concept of Yin and Yang as the two opposing forces of nature in the universe.

Yin is feminine, passive, centripetal (developing inward, proceeding toward the center).

Yang is masculine, positive, centrifugal (directed outward from the center).

With each going in a different direction you can see they *are* in opposition. And if you think it's a bother to count calories or carbohydrate grams, just try keeping track of Yin-Yang balance in your diet with no way to measure it!

The followers of Macrobiotics get around that technicality by eating the one single food which they believe contains the perfect balance of 5 parts Yin to 1 part Yang.

That food is rice. But you have to take it on faith. Only

skeptics ask who figured out the Yin-Yang ratio, and nobody knows the answer.

The mysticism of Macrobiotics seems to hold a special appeal for certain segments of our society. Today's young generation, with its growing interest in Eastern and Oriental philosophies, is responsible for much of the diet's renewed popularity. It's partly their patronage that has boosted the business of Yin-Yang restaurants in New York, Hollywood and San Francisco, where they can often see the swamis and yogis they admire.

Articles on the rice diet and its followers have appeared in many national magazines. The following popular version of the diet is the one that has proved the most harmful.

Breakfast, lunch and dinner—a bowl of unsalted rice.

Total daily liquid intake—½ cup of water and 1 cup of Bancha (or green) tea.

That's it. All of it. One self-styled authority says that if you don't drink that first sip of water in the morning you can do without it the rest of the day and night and not even miss it.

Maybe *you* won't miss it, but your body will.

Veteran fight fans will remember the defeat of Sugar Ray Robinson at Yankee Stadium some years ago when he tried a water-restricted, salt-free diet before weighing in for the match. The combination of salt and water restriction and a weight loss owing to dehydration sapped his strength and cost him the fight.

Induced dehydration puts a severe strain on the heart and other vital organs. It leaves the body a pound or two lighter, but lacking in muscle tone and feeling drained and exhausted.

If the cups are standard size, the 1½ cups of liquid allowed on the diet add up to 12 ounces a day. For normal function, the body requires *at least* 52 fluid ounces a day, which is about the amount it gives off daily. Since the body replenishes less than half of the fluids lost, the remainder must be supplied daily by liquids in the diet.

Water constitutes 85 percent of the gray matter of the brain and more than 90 percent of the blood plasma.

A loss of the body's water content can have serious effects on our blood's chemistry. A loss of only 10 percent can weaken the body and age the outward appearance by depriving the skin of moisture, causing it to dry and shrivel like an unwatered plant.

A loss of 20 to 22 percent can result in death.

Defenders of the rice diet will tell you of Dr. Walter Kempner and the diet program at Duke University, but Dr. Kempner himself says, "It's dangerous to go on a salt-free rice diet except under the kind of rigid supervision you get in the clinic."

Dr. Ohsawa justifies his Macrobiotics system by saying, "I take the position that every disease is produced by an excess in diet."

Some of them are, but not all. Just as many, or more, are produced by a *deficiency* in diet.

University of Pittsburgh's Dr. John F. Osterritter, in describing Dr. Ohsawa's diet in which "only one type of food (rice) was allowed for weeks and months," had this to say:

"Medically speaking, on a diet such as this, scurvy should appear in about three to five weeks. ... Several people starved to death on this diet."

Don't let it happen to *you!* Reduce safely on a diet that includes sufficient liquids and doesn't omit *any* of the essential nutrients.

8

If You Must *Crash Diet*

Crash diets in one form or another are here to stay, so the problem is not how to stop them (we can't!) but how to improve them.

Nutritionist Gaynor Maddox calls them "physically brutal, nutritionally reckless, psychologically ruthless"—and most of them are.

Yet every year an estimated 48 million persons go on them when they want to lose weight in a hurry. The trouble is, they don't keep it off. As soon as they stop dieting and go back to their old eating habits they start gaining again.

Sudden and drastic changes in the food intake can cause serious disturbances in the body mechanism of those who are no longer young. It can be dangerous not only for them, but for the anemic, the diabetic, or hypoglycemic of any age. If you belong to any of these groups, make a mental memo of three words that can mean the difference between a short life and a long one: NEVER CRASH DIET.

Those under forty and in good physical condition are usually able to withstand the punishment a crash diet inflicts on the body and still repair the damage done.

Yet sometimes even for them the repair is incomplete.

Whatever your age, a prolonged and drastically unbalanced diet can cause a loss of energy and vitality and lower your resistance to disease. It can make you nervous and irritable, change a good disposition to bad—and spoil a romance or marriage.

The best way to lose weight *permanently* is to lose it *slowly*.

77

Look at almost anyone who has lost too much too fast and you can see the aging effects of such a diet. When the skin loses its under-plumping layer of fat too rapidly to adjust, it collapses into loose, leftover folds that are especially noticeable underneath the chin and around the jawline.

A slower weight loss—say a pound or two a week on a high-protein diet—gives the skin a chance to tighten, prevents sagging and loss of muscle tone, and keeps you looking and feeling younger.

Still determined to go on a crash diet?

Yes, I know there are times when it comes in handy as an emergency measure. For example, when your weight zooms up unexpectedly behind your back, or wherever it zooms, and you absolutely *must* lop off four pounds by the weekend.

Or maybe you're already on a diet and have been losing steadily. Then suddenly—with no warning—your weight loss stops. You haven't been cheating, but the scales won't budge. You glare at them and feel picked on, discriminated against, and ready to give up. Why should this happen to *you?*

It happens to nearly everybody sometime during a diet. You've reached a stubborn, unaccountable weight plateau. Your weight loss has leveled off, lost its momentum.

You'll start losing again when your body has time to adjust to its loss of fat and the shift in its fluid balance.

But at this point you don't believe it. To the tune of "I'll Never Love Again" you go around humming "I'll Never Lose Again." You have a diet-dropout look in your eyes, and at the drop of a fork you'll be off your diet and starting a reckless food binge. *Unless . . .*

Somebody who has survived the same discouraging scene tells you that a day or two of crash dieting can get you past this impasse and on the road to Slimsville again. And it can.

Losing a few pounds quickly gives you the incentive to keep on losing. It works whether you're just beginning a diet or in the middle of one, stranded on a weight plateau engulfed in self-pity.

When a crash diet can do that it can't be *all* bad. Not for all the people. And not all the time. At least not if you choose it carefully and don't stay on it long without professional supervision.

Psychologically, many crash dieters are all-or-nothing individuals who can adapt to extreme measures but rebel at moderation. Their hang-up is that they prefer the temporary effects of a crash diet to a revision of their eating habits which would take weight off and keep it off.

Psychiatrist Hilde Bruch believes that some monotony in a crash diet is desirable because "it frees the dieter from thinking continuously of what he is going to eat next and of how to manipulate the diet. . . ." This seems particularly true of the all-or-nothing person, since he can cut *out* better than he can cut *down*.

Although Dr. Bruch disapproves of crash diets in general, she claims that limiting the food to a specific kind at any one meal is more effective than permitting a free choice among the allowed meats, fish, poultry, cheese, eggs and vegetables.

With that in mind, here is a limited but nutritious crash diet that is just as popular today as it was when it first appeared in 1956. Its originator, Ruth West, says, "You can take off not less than two pounds—and as much as five pounds, in *two* days," and she has thousands of successful dieters to back her up. It's still the most popular single diet of all time in Hollywood, where actors and actresses often have to slim down fast or lose a part.

A one-dish meal that requires almost no preparation, it fulfills Dr. Bruch's specifications for "effective monotony," and my own for meals high in protein and other balanced nutrients.

The Two-Day Cottage Cheese "Blitz" Diet
(Lelord Kordel version)

Basically, this diet is the same as Miss West's 1956 version except for two changes. I have substituted fresh fruit and/or raw vegetables for the artificially sweetened canned fruit of the original diet, and a drizzle of honey replaces the sugar she allowed at each meal.

Breakfast, lunch and dinner are the same; the only difference is in a variation of the fruits and vegetables.

Each meal consists of:

1 cup (8 ounces) of cottage cheese
Choice of low-carbohydrate fruit or raw vegetable

2 squares of Norwegian flatbread or Ry-Crisp
(brushed *lightly* with butter, drizzled with honey,
dusted with cinnamon and toasted under the
broiler)
Coffee or tea, no cream or sugar

The all-or-nothing person may prefer the same fruit or
vegetable for each meal, but if you like more variety, as I
do, choose any of these:

Breakfast—Choice of one:

Small orange, tangerine, fresh peach, 2 apricots,
small pear, 2 plums, nectarine, ½ grapefruit, ¾ cup of
strawberries or other fresh berries, half a small cantaloupe or a cup of assorted melon balls.

Luncheon and Dinner—Choice of the above fruits or
your favorite combination of these raw sliced or
shredded vegetables: tomato, cucumber, radishes,
celery, lettuce, watercress, carrot, zucchini, cauliflower, cabbage, chives, green onions or onion rings.

The charming, nutrition-minded Princess Alexandra
Kropotkin calls cottage cheese the "perfect basis for a diet
which will leave you feeling peppy and well fed." You
might like to try it the way she ate it as a child in Russia,
when garden vegetables were out of season.

"In winter we garnished our cottage cheese (*tvorog*)
with lightly fermented cabbage and apples," says the princess, "also with our Northern lingonberries. Russians consider cottage cheese the perfect health food—an absolute
daily necessity . . . on *any* sort of diet."

(See other diet suggestions by Princess Kropotkin in
Chapter 10, "Diets, Italian, Scandinavian, and Russian
Style").

Another Two-Day Cheese Diet

This is a favorite of actress Barbara Rush, who says she
can lose 5 pounds on it in two days. She and many of her
friends swear by it, but they admit that it should *never be
followed longer than 48 hours.*

Here, in Barbara's own words, is the diet:

*"You may have an unpeeled apple and natural cheese
as often as you wish all day long."*
Yes, it's monotonous—but only for two days.
Black, unsweetened coffee and tea are allowed.

The *New* Bananas-and-Skim-Milk Diet

The old bananas-and-skim-milk diet of some years ago
consisted of two bananas and a glass of skim milk three
times a day. That was all. It was popular for quite a
while, especially among the all-or-nothing dieters. But
even they soon tired of the diet and its popularity died.
Luckily, it expired before the dieters did.

Now a new, less monotonous and far more nutritious
version of the diet has appeared.

Breakfast and luncheon are the same as those of the old
diet—two bananas and a glass of skim milk for each
meal. It's the dinner menu that breaks the monotony and
changes a substandard diet to one that's acceptable, at
least for a few days at a time.

The dinner menu allows you:

> ½ broiled chicken (don't eat the skin!)
> ¾ cup steamed broccoli
> 15 medium mushroom buttons
> ½ bunch watercress
> 1 rye cracker
> 1 tbsp cottage cheese
> 1 cup skim milk
> 1 ripe banana, fresh or broiled
> Black coffee or tea

Certainly the dinner is more than adequate. But to
make it nutritionally more desirable, I would recommend
adding more salad greens and raw vegetables to the watercress. And who wants *another* banana after stuffing them
down all day? Instead, have some other fresh fruit of your
choice. It will break the monotony, but not your weight
loss. Bananas were chosen for this diet because they are
more *filling* than other fruits, not because they are less
fattening.

These diets are examples of the monotony that Dr.
Bruch and others consider desirable in a short-term crash

diet. All of them have succeeded in the majority of cases, partly because they *are* monotonous and easy to follow. When you eat the same thing meal after meal you soon lose your appetite for it and eat less and less. That's one of its advantages in taking off weight. It's also one of its dangers, if you stay on it long. Unless a crash diet is carefully planned, it can rob you of a whopping percent of the nutrients you need just to keep breathing.

Before she crash-dieted her way into a hospital, a 19-year-old girl once told me, "It doesn't matter what I'm eating less of if I can lose weight on it!"

But it *does* matter, as actress Carol Lynley found out when she was a teen-ager. You can reduce on ice cream and black coffee three times a day and endanger your health, as she did. Or you can lose weight quickly but *safely* on the high-protein, semirestricted diet that follows.

Lelord Kordel's Choose-Your-Protein Diet

Breakfast:

To get the most nutritional mileage out of the least amount of food compatible with health, breakfast is practically the same every day. All-or-nothing types may prefer to keep all their meals exactly the same, but a limited choice is offered for those who want it.

Choice of one: ½ grapefruit, a small orange or tangerine, or 4 oz of unsweetened grapefruit juice.

Choice of: 2 eggs (may be cooked any way you like in a pan lightly brushed with safflower oil, but no butter)

or

1 egg and 2 tablespoons of cottage cheese or a wedge of cheddar, Swiss or other natural cheese.

Black coffee, coffee substitute, tea and herb teas without sugar are allowed at each meal and between meals, as desired.

Luncheon and Dinner:

You may start each meal with hot or jellied bouillon or consommé, or have them any other time of day you like. For an entrée, choose your favorite protein food from the following list, cooked any way except fried.

Choice of one: Hamburger, beef, lamb, veal, liver, or other organ meats.
Chicken or turkey, with skin removed.
Fresh fish and seafood, or canned salmon, tuna, sardines, crabmeat, lobster or shrimp.
1 leafy green or combination salad with safflower oil and vinegar dressing.

The first few days of this diet will usually show no weight loss, but by the end of the week an average person will suddenly drop from three to five pounds.

Some calcium is provided by the leafy greens in the salad, but if you stay on it longer than a week add two glasses of skim milk, buttermilk, or a cup of cottage cheese a day.

If you *must* crash diet be sure it's one that doesn't impair your health, interfere with your daily activities, or unbalance your budget. A diet that derails you physically, socially, psychologically or economically is not for you, no matter how well it works for others.

I know a writer who can lose several pounds in a week by eating normally during the day, but having only champagne, caviar and truffles for dinner. It works for him, but not everybody would like it—or could afford it.

Remember that even the best crash diet should be no more than a temporary emergency measure.

You can only get slim and *stay* slim on a balanced diet that you can live with and not feel frustrated and deprived. One that suits your taste, temperament, and way of life, and reduces you slowly but *safely*.

9

Fasting to Break the
Pound Barrier

After two chapters dealing with the extremes of dieting, it's with some misgivings that I now turn to one on fasting.

Yet I have purposely written this chapter to follow the others to avoid any misunderstanding that might arise concerning it. The previous chapters stressed the importance of eating a balanced diet at all times, whether you're dieting or not.

This one explains some of the advantages of *not* eating for brief periods.

Dr. Edgar S. Gordon, of the University of Wisconsin Medical School, is one of an increasing number of doctors who recommend a 48-hour fast before beginning a diet.

"The aim," says Dr. Gordon, "is not to produce any spectacular weight loss, but rather to break the existing metabolic pattern."

I know from personal experience what an occasional fast of short duration does for me, and from experiments and observation what it can do for others.

I have watched its effectiveness at the beginning of a diet and in the middle of one, where it can break the pound barrier of a weight plateau by getting the stalled weight-shedding process started again.

But notice that I said a fast *of short duration*. A do-it-yourself fast should not be longer than two or three days, *and only those who are in good physical condition should attempt it without professional supervision.*

When You Should *Not* Fast

Common sense should send out this warning to anyone with a gastric or duodenal ulcer who is on frequent feedings: "No fasting for you!"

The same is true of the person with high blood sugar (diabetes) or low blood sugar (hypoglycemia or hyperinsulinism) and, although they are seldom overweight, those with Addison's disease.

The metabolic character of some reducing diets and fasts may produce undesirable side effects in anyone with cirrhosis of the liver or gout. There is some evidence that long-term or total fasting can produce gout, as there is a continuing production of uric acid due to cellular breakdown.

Superobese persons (those who have up to 100 pounds or more to lose) may develop both physical and emotional complications during a fast. When a prolonged fast is prescribed for them, as it often is, they are sent to a hospital for what is called "therapeutic starvation." There they are under strict supervision, where any adverse reactions can be checked.

In the metabolic ward of Loyola University's Stritch School of Medicine, a Chicago physician, Dr. David S. Swanson, recorded the psychological reactions of patients weighing over 300 pounds. He found that in these patients food produced a genial lethargy, drowsiness, and freedom from stress known as the Pickwickian syndrome (from the characterization of the fat boy in Dickens' *Pickwick Papers*).

Before the fast they were friendly, pleasant and relaxed. But when food was withheld from them they brooded, became tense, quarrelsome, suspicious and depressed. For many superobese, eating is an escape from their suppressed frustrations. Deprive them of food and their hidden emotional disturbances come to the surface.

"It varies from individual to individual," says Dr. Swanson. "It is not a paranoia or a severe neurosis. It is something distinctly unpleasant which they feel unable to cope with. So they eat much like the alcoholic who drinks."

If you belong in any of these categories or have other

*health or emotional problems, be sure to get professional
advice before going on any kind of fast.*

But if your health is good . . .

If you aren't grossly overweight . . .

If you're neither a child nor a senior citizen . . .

You may find that from one to three days of fasting
can make you look and feel better than you have in years.

It can, as Dr. Gordon said, break the existing metabolic
pattern (and the pound barrier!), decrease your appetite
by resetting your appestat and "shrinking" your stomach,
and make it easier for you to lose weight faster. It can be
a detoxifying process that makes your mind and body
more alert, gives you a younger, clearer skin, and promotes a general sense of mental and physical well-being.

There are many ways of fasting. Since ancient times,
total fasting has meant abstaining from all food and drink
except water. It was prescribed by early Greek physicians,
including the great Hippocrates and Galen. Plato, Soc-
rates, and other renowned thinkers of their time went on
occasional fasts "to attain mental and physical efficiency."

Students of the Bible will remember the fasts of Christ,
Moses, Elijah, and David, some of which lasted forty days
and nights.

Centuries passed, but the habit of fasting remained.
Paracelsus, a Swiss physician and alchemist of the sixteenth
century, called fasting "the greatest remedy . . . the
physician within," and many modern European doctors
agree. One of Germany's leading fast specialists, Professor
Werner Zabel, M.D., expresses my own opinion on the
subject when he says, "Together . . . *with optimal nutrition,* fasting is man's oldest healing method." (My italics.)

But today the total fasting of ancient times is seldom
practiced except in clinics and hospitals, and by the few
remaining hardy souls who have iron wills and constitu-
tions to match.

A friend of mine who has both considers me overly
cautious in warning older persons against going on either a
total or an unsupervised fast. He is Paul Bragg, noted
physical therapist, writer and lecturer, who has had more
than fifty years personal experience with fasting.

Now in his nineties and a great-grandfather, Paul belongs to hiking, dancing, tennis, swimming and mountain-
climbing clubs, and is active in all of them. When he

lectures in Hawaii he never misses a chance to go surfing and hula dancing, which he does as expertly as the natives.

A few months ago we had dinner in Honolulu, and although I have long been familiar with his nutritional way of life, he told me in a single sentence what he believes to be his greatest secret of health, youthful energy, and a strong, slender body.

"I believe in short fasts," he said, *"with good nutrition and good living habits between fasts."*

Paul, who calls himself a "health billionaire," goes on a 24- to 36-hour fast every week of his life. In addition, he fasts for a week or more at regular intervals four times a year—spring, summer, fall and winter. But he knows his own body and its requirements and is quick to recognize when his fasts should begin and end. Since he conditioned himself to this régime during his youth, he is an exception to the rule that applies to others over sixty or to anyone with chronic or degenerative disabilities:

"No total fasting without professional supervision."

The modern and most popular form of fasting, both in Europe and America, is the modified or semifast. It consists of water and either fresh vegetable or fruit juices, or both. Most of them also allow herb teas, bouillon, strained vegetable broth, and if you *must,* an occasional cup of black, unsweetened coffee.

Several days of this type of fasting have proved safe and beneficial for persons in normal health. Except in abnormal cases, dieters on a short, modified fast lose just as much weight as those on a total fast. And they do it easily, with little or no discomfort.

The reducing benefits of a fast have been described by *Vogue* magazine in these words: "To lose weight fast, you have to *fast*—just cut down your intake of food to the vanishing point."

But what about the health benefits? What actually happens to the body temporarily released from the daily burden of digesting large quantities of food?

We know that it's a natural instinct of animals to fast when sick or wounded. Nature wisely helps them along by removing their desire for food and suspending the senses of taste and smell.

During a fast, all the forces of the body released from

food digestion are concentrated on healing and the elimination of toxins.

As the body burns up the useless fat deposits—often with large amounts of impurities embedded in them—an internal cleansing and detoxification begins. The expendable fat and diseased or damaged tissues are burned first, leaving the vital tissues intact.

A German doctor, Otto H. F. Buchinger, Jr., M.D., calls fasting "a burning of rubbish." Dr. Buchinger, who is known in Europe as "the champion of therapeutic fasting in modern times," has found that fasting increases the cleansing capacity of the eliminative organs (kidneys, liver, lungs and skin) so they can expel toxins and metabolic wastes with greater speed and efficiency.

Fasting gives the digestive and protective organs a rest. The stomach and intestines, relieved of their usual tasks of dealing with food, can start clearing away mucus deposits and other toxic accumulations.

For the cleansing benefits of vinegar, and the energy values of honey and safflower oil, and to prevent hunger pangs, I included formula HOV three times a day during my own two-day fast, and recommend it to others.

Some authorities on fasting suggest an enema before a fast and at regular intervals during one, but I don't advise it. On an all-liquid diet a lack of residue is to be expected. If constipation occurs, the condition will automatically correct itself in all but the most stubborn cases. But for those who feel the need of it, a mild herbal laxative is permissible.

Richard Condon, author of *The Manchurian Candidate* and *The Pleasures of Fasting,* says that you can become "hooked on fasting."

"Aside from the intense pleasure of seeing your excess pounds drop away," he says, "and your circulatory system shape up and your internal organs rest, there's a wonderful psychological benefit ... an odd biochemical change comes over the body. ... A chemical called ethanol is formed in the system. It's similar to watered alcohol and causes the faster to get quite a buzz on."

Condon doesn't say how the buzz affects him on his annual two-week's fast, but he continues with this observation: "All the great religious leaders who were supposed to be caught up in an ecstasy of religious exaltation ... actually, they were stoned!"

Whether you want to reduce, improve your health and appearance, or "get a buzz on," here are some fasting suggestions that can be easily adapted for home use.

Elizabeth Arden's famous—and expensive!—Maine Chance starts its reducing program with this preliminary cleansing fast:

Every two hours—a glass of fresh vegetable or fruit juice.

Three times a day—a cup of strained vegetable broth made of carrots, celery, string beans, parsley, mushrooms and watercress.

For protein, an egg is beaten into the cup of strained broth while it's still hot enough to coddle the egg.

Alan H. Nittler, M.D., an authority on detoxifying diets, puts his patients on a three-day fast of freshly prepared carrot juice and other fresh vegetable juices, plus vitamins. Organically grown vegetables should be used, if possible. If not, they should be thoroughly scrubbed to remove all traces of pesticide sprays.

If you don't have a juicer to liquefy raw vegetables, Dr. Nittler suggests either of these alternatives:

1. As much grapefruit and celery as you like, any time you want them. (You aren't likely to gorge yourself on either!) Water is the allowed beverage.

2. For his second alternative, Dr. Nittler recommends a fast that has been popular in European health and reducing spas for many years. Known as the European Grape Cure, it consists of nothing but fresh grapes and water.

In European spas, medically supervised grape diets begin with no more than two ounces of grapes a meal for the first day. Each day the portion is increased, until by the fourth or fifth day the patient may have up to three or four pounds a day.

Dr. Nittler limits his fasts to three days, and during that time he says you may have as much of the specified juices or food as you like, whenever you feel hungry. In his opinion, vegetable juices are more desirable than the alternate fasts. I agree with him, although I would put it more strongly. Almost anyone in good health can benefit from a short fast on vegetable or fruit juices, *but . . .*

Too many persons are not able to handle the large amounts of certain elements in the alternate diets—the citric acid in grapefruit, the roughage of celery, and even such natural sugar as that of grapes.

All of them are excellent foods in moderation, but not as a total diet. At least not for three days without the physical checkup and close supervision that Dr. Nittler gives his patients.

If you have none of the problems above or those listed on page 77, you might try either of the alternate fasts for a maximum of one day, or for a meal or two a day, until you can judge your reaction to them. And if you choose the grape fast, be sure the grapes are ripe and well-washed, eat them slowly and chew them well.

Dr. Kurt Donsbach is another expert who has had great success with the following three-day liquid fast and detoxifier, which he originated for his own patients.

1st day: Put through the juicer enough fresh, raw beets, tops and all, to make 2 fluid ounces. Mix with two quarts of water, add the juice of a dozen lemons and sweeten to taste with honey. Drink at desired intervals to prevent hunger.

2nd day: Water, honey and lemon mixture the same as above, but this time liquefy enough beet roots and greens to make 4 fluid ounces.

3rd day: Same as the second day, except that you add 2 additional fluid ounces of beets and greens for a total of 6 ounces.

I have personally tried Dr. Donsbach's fast and have recommended it to my clients, not only for reducing, but as a good source of vitamins, iron and calcium, as an internal cleanser and liver detoxifier.

The majority of weight-conscious stage and screen celebrities go on regular, semiregular or occasional fasts. "If you can spend a couple of days on lemon juice and hot water," says June Allyson, "it will clear out the toxins."

Not recommended for everybody, but June's petite figure, glowing complexion and vitality are proof that it works for her.

The legendary Mae West, who at 77 weighs a well-distributed 123 pounds, is a regular one-day-a-week faster. "I squeeze the juice from six oranges, three grapefruit and two lemons," she says. "Then I add an equal amount of distilled water. I fast all day on that."

Van Johnson is another one-day-a-week faster, sometimes on juices, often on nothing but water. "For a cleaner-outer," he says.

And as a slimmer-downer and weight controller.

Singer Lena Horne and actresses Rhonda Fleming and Jean Simmons fast one day a month on fresh fruit and vegetable juices.

The daily diet of Jean and her family consists largely of organically grown fresh fruits, vegetables, meat and poultry from California health-food stores. "I don't go along with the way food is treated now," she says, "with all the additives and sprays."

Here is how she makes what she calls "a very good health drink," which she enjoys whether she is fasting or not.

"You shove a mixture of carrots, celery, parsley, green peppers, apples or anything else you want into a juice-arator," is the way Jean describes it. "You can make it sweeter by adding peaches if you like. Either way it tastes delicious . . . and it's a marvelous energizer."

Actor James Coburn, tall, lean and muscular, goes to the desert alone for occasional periods of fasting that keep him physically fit and mentally refreshed. He believes with James Condon and many creative and professional persons that fasting can be a rewarding psychological experience.

Playwright, novelist, and political and social critic Gore Vidal explained his return from the Island of Ischia this way: "I frequently go off to retreats for several days to fast, lose weight, meditate, and get a lot of reading done." And perhaps, as other dedicated and thinking men have done, to reach new heights of mental and spiritual realization?

The following fast-and-diet regime is based on the theory that almost anyone can fast or stay on a restricted diet for two days at a time. The constantly changing pace of the two-by-two reducing plan makes the most of the dieter's initial enthusiasm, prevents monotony, gets him off to a fast weight loss that reinforces his willpower and keeps him from backsliding.

The Australian Two-By-Two Fast *and* Diet

(Lelord Kordel variation)

The basic changes of food pattern every two days are the same in my version as those of the original. The variations have been made because of the difference in American tastes and to insure optimum nutrition.

In Australia, the food for each day is made up of set menus, with no substitutions. Mine is a take-your-choice variation that gives you a selection of your favorite foods within the named categories, with a nutritional plus or two included in all of them.

To provide sufficient vitamins, minerals, and enzymes on the fasting days, I have substituted your choice of fresh vegetable or fruit juices for their marmite (a warm drink made of vegetable extract).

First Two Days: Liquids Only—*Plus*

Two days of fasting start your diet, but are not repeated unless you hit a weight plateau and stop losing. If that happens, go back on liquids for another two days.

Take your choice of the fasts already mentioned, preferably fresh vegetable or fruit juices, strained vegetable broth, bouillon, herb teas, and if you can't get along without it, black unsweetened coffee.

The Australian version allows a pint of milk a day except on the protein days, when it's cut to ½ pint. For a faster weight loss and as a cholesterol discourager for adults, I advise skim milk or buttermilk.

PLUS: my nutritional plus on fasting days is a tablespoon of brewer's yeast flakes dissolved in a glass of vegetable juice or skim milk twice a day.

Water whenever you want it on all the two-by-two days. And formula HOV is a good addition to any of them.

Second Two Days: Vegetables and Fruits—*Plus*

These two days will break your fast gently and prepare your stomach for the protein meals to follow.

Choose your favorite low-carbohydrate vegetables from the list on pages 191-2, and remember you can eat all you want of them. Have them in salads with safflower oil and vinegar or lightly cooked in a minimum of water.

Since I have a habit of trying a diet myself before recommending it, I've been asked repeatedly what fruits and vegetables I ate and what I did about breakfast.

Nobody seems to have any trouble choosing their favorite juices and broths for fasting, or food for the protein days. But for these two days they want examples, so here are the lists I chose from. Most of the vegetables are on the Eat-All-You-Want list, but a few are not. During this part of the diet I ate an average of ten to twelve low-carbohydrate vegetables and four fruits a day.

VEGETABLES

Asparagus	Eggplant
Beans, green	Green peppers
Bean sprouts	Lettuce
Beet greens	Mushrooms
Cabbage	Mustard greens
Cauliflower	Romaine
Carrots	Spinach
Celery	Summer squash
Chard	Turnip greens
Chinese cabbage	Tomatoes
Cucumber	Watercress
Dandelion greens	Zucchini

PLUS: 1. (To keep from going completely vegetarian) One or two eggs cooked any way except fried.

PLUS: 2. A cup of cottage cheese or yogurt may be substituted for one cup of the daily milk allowance.

FRUITS

Blackberries (½ cup)	Papaya (½ cup, diced)
Cantaloupe (½ med.)	Peach (1 med.)
Grapefruit (½ med.)	Plums (2)
Honeydew melon (2-inch slice)	Raspberries (½ cup)
	Strawberries (1 cup)
Muskmelon (½ med.)	Tangerine (1 med.)
Nectarine (1 small)	

You want to know why apples aren't on the list? They aren't as high in carbohydrate as nectarines, and they're a fine, healthful food—except for fatties.

It's been found that the pectin in apples tends to hold fluids in the body. Useful in war if no blood plasma is available, but it's a handicap in the war against fat. So if you're easily waterlogged, you'll reduce faster by omitting apples until you're slim again.

You think you absolutely *can't* eat vegetables for breakfast, but you want more than just fruit, so what can you do?

I don't believe in starting the day with a skimpy meal, either. That's why I added two proteins as the plus foods on these two days, but don't sell vegetables for breakfast short until you've tried them. Here's what I had:

Breakfast   *1st day*

　½ grapefruit
　2 eggs scrambled with mushrooms, chopped green
　　pepper and zucchini
　　　　　　　　2nd day
　Strawberries drizzled lightly with honey and orange
　　juice
　Poached eggs on a nest of beet greens (or spinach)
　2 or 3 slices each of tomato and eggplant, broiled or
　　grilled

Luncheon   *1st day*

　Consommé or bouillon
　Large leafy green salad with safflower oil and cider
　　vinegar
　Choice of fruit for dessert
　Cup of herb tea or glass of buttermilk
　　　　　　　　2nd day
Same as above, except that each day I varied my choice
of salad greens and fruit.

Dinner   *1st day*

　Choice of any clear soup or 4 ounces of tomato juice
　Cottage cheese (the second *plus* food of the day)
　A vegetable-*plus* plate, with a favorite selection of
　　fresh vegetables, both cooked and raw, surround-
　　ing the mound of protein-rich cottage cheese
　Choice of fruit for dessert
　Choice of beverage, no cream or sugar
　　　　　　　　2nd day
Same as above except for a different choice of vegeta-
bles and fruits.

Third Two Days: Protein Only—*Plus*

Chapter 7 explained the dangers of omitting either fats, protein, or carbohydrates from the diet for any length of time. But when you alternate two days of fruits and vegetables with two days of protein you don't omit any of them.

Within each four-day period you're getting all the essential food elements and maintaining a good weekly balance of them.

The vegetable and fruit days supply the necessary carbohydrates, vitamins, minerals and enzymes. Protein and fat are provided on the alternate days.

For the two protein days take your choice of the following foods, *but absolutely nothing else:*

Lean beef, veal, organ meats, poultry, fish, seafood, eggs, natural, unprocessed cheese, and cottage, farmer or pot cheese.

PLUS foods: 2 stalks of celery, 1 cucumber, and 10 mushrooms. Not enough carbohydrate to count in any of them, and they do add flavor and variety to an all-protein menu.

Drink a minimum of eight glasses of water a day. Have bouillon, consommé and black, unsweetened coffee and tea, as desired. *No soft drinks—not even the no-cal type.* Yes, I know what you've been told. But the sodium carbonate in them, like salt, retains fluids in the body and waterlogs the tissues.

The resulting edema weighs as much and looks as hefty as plain old fat. To lose both of them faster, cut down on salt and cut out carbonated beverages.

After the first two days of fasting, Australians alternate between the two protein days and the two vegetable and fruit days for as long as they need to lose weight. The two-by-twos have become something of a classic in their country, and they're about the healthiest looking people I've ever seen!

The changing rhythm every two days prevents chemical or "hidden" hunger, keeps you feeling satisfied so you aren't tempted to cheat, and results in a steady weight loss.

The famous Buchinger Clinic in Bad Pyrmont, Germany, is directed by the same Dr. Buchinger you met earlier in the chapter.

There, under his guidance and that of his associates, more than 70,000 patients have fasted successfully.

One of them was a New York model, Susan Schönborn, who went there to lose the pounds she had gained during a holiday in Greece. Susan had what she called "real solid fat to break down," which is the hardest kind to lose. But after three weeks at the clinic she returned to New York looking sensational, her skin firm, clear and glowing—and ten pounds thinner.

When Susan described her Buchinger fast, she might have been speaking of the one I use and have recommended for years. But coming from a world-famous clinic on the beautiful shores of Lake Constance, it sounds impressive and glamorous (even to me!).

Here, in Susan's own words, is how she fasted:

"I had nothing for the first two weeks but vegetable bouillon and fresh vegetable juices—tomato, celery, carrot—plus one spoonful of honey every day. Very little salt at lunchtime, none at dinner."

After two weeks of liquids, Susan's fast was broken with the addition of yogurt and fresh fruit compotes, and a gentle transition to solid foods began.

At the Buchinger clinic and other reducing spas, fasters are under continual expert supervision. A long fast should never be undertaken without it. But two or three days on fresh fruit and vegetable juices is safe if you're in good physical and emotional health. And here are just a few of the benefits that you can expect from it:

1. The digestive apparatus and pancreas are given a rest and digestive upsets are relieved.

2. Acting as an internal cleanser and "burner of rubbish," fasting rids the body of toxins and impurities.

3. It can clear a dull, blemished complexion and revive the fresh, youthful beauty of the skin.

4. It can improve your circulatory system, take a load off your heart, and increase your mental awareness.

5. And finally, it can break the pound barrier, get you past a discouraging weight plateau, and give you the incentive to keep on losing.

If you decide that fasting is compatible with your health, age, and way of life, remember this:

Make them short, modified fasts of fresh vegetable and fruit juices, *with good nutrition and good living habits between fasts.*

10

Diets: Italian, Scandinavian, and Russian Style

The Italian diet came, logically enough, from Rome; and that's where I was when I heard of it. When it was first described to me it sounded so much like the diets I usually recommend that I didn't try to get a copy of it.

I didn't have to try. Almost every Italian I knew insisted that I should have it and told me how sensational it was. A charming journalist friend of mine, Rina Andolfo, didn't just tell me. She showed me.

Gesturing toward them as though I didn't know where they were, she said, "You know my Italian hips?"

"Let's put it another way," I said. "I recognize them when you're wearing them. And they look fine on you."

"Ah, maybe now, since the diet! But before they were so heavy, so *Italian* I couldn't get rid of them and had to hide them with full skirts." Proudly she smoothed the narrow skirt over her hips and turned around so I could admire them from all angles.

I did. And found every angle admirable. "Would you mind twirling around again?" I asked.

"So!" she laughed. "Now you change your mind and take the diet back to America with you?"

"You've convinced me," I admitted. "I wouldn't leave Italy without it."

It was originated by Wolfgang Goetz-Claren of Rome, who believes that a diet should start with a régime to detoxify the body. The first three days of his diet is limited to fruits and vegetables only.

If you think that it sounds like the three-day fasting

program, you're right. And some of his basic diet rules will also sound familiar to you. Here they are:

1. All food must be fresh, and some should be eaten raw.

2. Use as little salt as possible, and sea salt is preferable. Let herbs, garlic and freshly ground black pepper compensate for the lack of salt.

3. No white sugar. When you must have sweetening, use natural, unprocessed honey.

4. No bread. One of the thin wafers of Norwegian flatbread is allowed for each meal, if desired.

5. You may have a cup of consommé, bouillon, or strained vegetable broth before luncheon and dinner, or between meals. Fresh vegetable juices may also be taken as midmorning or midafternoon snacks.

6. No commercial salad dressings and no mayonnaise. Safflower oil, olive or other vegetable oil, and vinegar or lemon may be used as a salad dressing. If you like, season it to taste with grated onion, a crushed garlic clove, paprika and mustard, blending until smooth.

7. No coffee or milk. Allowed drinks are tea with lemon, all the herb teas you want, and moderate amounts of fresh vegetable juices.

8. A 4-ounce glass of dry red or white wine is allowed for luncheon and dinner, *on fish and meat days only*.

9. For dessert you may have your choice of a small orange, ½ grapefruit, a tangerine, or a small pear or peach.

Dr. Goetz-Claren calls his diet "a gourmet approach to health and slimming," and my Italian friends assure me that they lose from 3 to 5 pounds a week on it, never get hunger pangs and don't get tired of the food, which renews their energy as pasta never could.

The Italian 12-Day Regeneration Diet

Breakfast is the same every day, Muesli and tea with lemon. And although Muesli is made of oatmeal, which is usually restricted on diets, and apples, which we now know tend to retain fluid in the tissues of some persons, Dr. Goetz-Claren says that in this combination they aren't fattening.

Muesli, developed by the great Dr. Bircher-Benner of Switzerland, is made of *raw* oatmeal, and the experts claim that it's only fattening when cooked. There are many variations of Muesli, some made with raw steel-cut oats, others with the old-fashioned rolled variety, but never with the quick-cooking or instant variety. The original recipe also contained chopped hazelnuts and raisins, but for dieters here is the recipe Dr. Goetz-Claren uses and recommends:

MUESLI
(1 serving)

Soak 1 tablespoon of raw oatmeal overnight in enough water to cover. The next morning stir in 1 teaspoon each of lemon juice and honey and top with 1 unpeeled grated apple.

(Ready-to-eat Muesli is now available in most health food stores for those who want a quick, easy breakfast.)

1st day

Lunch: Two eggs, any style
              Any vegetable salad
Dinner: Broiled mushrooms
              Spinach

2nd day

Lunch: Any fruit salad
Dinner: Vegetable plate

3rd day

Lunch: Salad of greens, tomatoes, raisins
Dinner: Two eggs, any style
              Any vegetable

4th day

Lunch: Chicken salad (mixed with oil and vinegar
              —no mayonnaise)
Dinner: Salmon
              Broccoli or equal vegetable

5th day

Lunch: Sweetbreads or liver (sautéed in butter or
            oil—add sherry if desired)
Dinner: Steak (8 oz) grilled or broiled
            Spinach lightly cooked *or*
            Spinach and chopped-onion salad

6th day

Lunch: Crab and cucumber salad
Dinner: Any fowl
            Any salad

7th day

Lunch: Any fruit salad
Dinner: Two eggs, any style
            One vegetable
            Green salad

8th day

Lunch: Any vegetable salad
Dinner: Two lamb chops (fat removed)
            One vegetable
            Sliced tomatoes

9th day

Lunch: Hamburger, grilled, broiled, or sautéed
            Green salad
Dinner: Any white fish
            Any salad

10th day

Lunch: Shrimp salad
Dinner: Calf's tongue (hot or cold)
            Two vegetables

11th day

Lunch: Two eggs, any style
            One small ground-beef patty
Dinner: Any meat except pork
            Any two vegetables

12th day

Lunch: Any fruit salad
Dinner: Any fish
           Any two vegetables

Diets from Finland and Norway

In Finland, a lively young magazine called *Kaueneus ja Terveys* (*Beauty and Health*) keeps its readers informed on the newest and best diets.

The magazine's trim blond editor, Sirkka Keskinen, explains their editorial policy in three words: "We're *very* antifat!"

The following diet, approved by them and planned by a Finnish physician, starts with one day of modified fasting. Those who have tried it tell me that you can lose five pounds in five days on it. But don't stay on it longer than five days at a time and, for health insurance, take a vitamin-mineral supplement like Nutri-Time each day.

Finnish 5-Day Diet for a 5-Pound Weight Loss

1st day (Modified fasting)

Breakfast: Tea with honey
Luncheon: 1 apple
Dinner: 1 cup of vegetable broth

2nd day

Breakfast: Fresh prunes
              Rye wafers or Norwegian flatbread with
                 cottage cheese
              Tea with honey
Luncheon: Fresh vegetable juice
Dinner: Fresh fruit salad
              Wafers with cottage cheese
              Black coffee

3rd day

Breakfast: 1 orange
              Norwegian flatbread with cottage cheese
              Tea with honey

Luncheon:	Steamed carrots and brown rice
	Lettuce with lemon juice
	1 cup of yogurt
	Glass of buttermilk
Dinner:	Fresh fruit salad
	Wafers with cottage cheese
	Glass of skim milk or buttermilk

4th day

Breakfast:	1 slice pumpernickel bread, lightly buttered
	Tea with honey
Luncheon:	1 small baked potato topped with a table-spoon of cottage cheese (no butter)
	Steamed spinach or other leafy greens
	1 banana
	Glass of buttermilk
Dinner:	Steamed brown rice and tomatoes
	Choice of two or three fresh fruits
	Black coffee

5th day

Breakfast:	Fresh prunes
	Rye wafers with cottage cheese
	Tea with honey
Luncheon:	Raw vegetable salad
	Small baked potato with 1 pat of butter
	Choice of cheese and beverage
Dinner:	Steamed brown rice and tomatoes
	1 slice lightly buttered pumpernickel bread
	Choice of all the fresh fruit you want
	Black coffee

After five days, my advice is to start adding eggs, fish, and meat to your diet, substitute a citrus fruit for prunes, and omit the rice, bread, butter, and potatoes until you've slimmed down to your desired weight.

The Norwegian Alternating Diet

This diet, which first appeared in *Aftenpoften,* one of Oslo's leading newspapers, was given to me by an American correspondent in Norway and is similar to our own high-protein diets. Prunes and bananas seem to be standard fruits on all Scandinavian diets, perhaps because they don't have access to the wide variety of fresh fruits that Americans take for granted, both in and out of season.

No day-by-day menus are given for this diet. Except for breakfast, which is the same every day, you alternate between the two daily choices for luncheon and dinner. You may substitute other green vegetables and fresh fruits for those listed, but the alternating pattern of fish and meat should not be broken.

Breakfast: (Standard)

1 medium orange
1 boiled egg
2 slices of bacon
1 cup of black coffee

(In my opinion, bacon is too high in fat and too low in food value for dieters to waste their restricted food allowance on. If you don't want to omit it, you can render most of the fat out of it by simmering it in boiling water for ten minutes and patting it dry in a paper towel before broiling it.)

Luncheon:

Alternate between these two choices:

I

1 cup of yogurt
Black coffee

II

An open-face sandwich made with 1 slice of whole-grain bread topped with your choice of roast beef, tongue, liver pâté, shrimps, or sardines

Dinner:
Alternate between these two choices:

I

Broiled fish, any kind
Green beans (or other green vegetable)
Fresh prunes (or other fresh fruit)
Black coffee

II

Calf's liver with onions
Cauliflower (or broccoli, cabbage, leafy greens or
    other low-carbohydrate vegetable)
1 tomato
1 banana (or choice of other fresh fruit)
Black coffee

The alternating diet combines sound nutrition with what
I am told is a rapid weight loss of from five to ten pounds
within two weeks.

The Russian Fish and Cottage-Cheese Diet

This diet follows the general pattern of one originated
by Princess Alexandra Kropotkin, and contains the same
amount of cottage cheese that she recommends.

Breakfast:
    ½ grapefruit
    1 egg cooked any way except fried
    1 slice cracked wheat or rye bread spread with
        2 tablespoons cottage cheese
    Black, unsweetened coffee or tea

Luncheon:
    Large leafy green salad with safflower oil and vinegar
        dressing
    5 tablespoons cottage cheese
    2 rye wafers
    1 medium apple
    Black, unsweetened coffee or tea

Dinner:

    Choice of any kind of fish or seafood, with lemon and horseradish dressing

    1 small baked potato, seasoned with paprika, minced watercress and chopped chives

    Sliced beets and cucumbers, marinated in cider vinegar

    5 tablespoons cottage cheese topped with ½ cup of lingonberries and grated orange peel

Breakfast is the same every day, but by varying the vegetables and fruit to avoid monotony and by substituting meat for fish two or three days a week, you may stay on the diet as long as necessary to normalize your weight. According to my information, you should lose between three and four pounds a week. Probably more if you substituted a leafy green vegetable for the baked potato and omitted the bread.

Alexei A. Pokrovsky, director of the Institute of Nourishment of the Soviet Academy of Medical Science and an expert on diet, says, "we like bread very much in our country. And we have some very fat ladies and gentlemen."

Pokrovsky emphasizes a diet of natural foods, with nothing canned or processed. He recommends meals based on protein-rich foods, lean meat, nonfat milk and cottage cheese, and a total food intake of no more than 2,000 calories a day. It's his belief that "diet is the urgent problem of our day," and he gives lectures on proper diet and daily exercise to the news media, on radio programs, and to school, factory, and business groups.

"We have gotten used to too much food," he warns, especially high-caloric food, and must change our diet if we want to be healthy, do better work, stay slim and strong and live longer."

He advises Soviet women to use vegetable oils for their family's health and for complexion beauty. "And avoid sweets," he says. "Sweets are the most dangerous, perfidious enemy of women."

His latest pride is a nutritional development called belip. An all-purpose protein food used successfully by dieters, belip is popular with nondieters, too. It's made of fish, curds, and vegetable oils, but I was unable to get the recipe during my brief visit to Russia.

After trying to buy belip in several Moscow stores, I was told it was available at a diet store at the foot of Gorki street. When I found the place and told the clerk what I wanted, she said, "No more. Every store in Moscow all sold out."

Production had stopped temporarily, she said, because the factory was out of some "secret ingredients" and was waiting for them to arrive. Perhaps on another trip to Russia I can find out more about belip, or bring some back to America for us to sample.

Until then, remember that belip consists largely of fish, curds (cottage cheese, yogurt, whey or kefir) and vegetable oils. Give these foods priority in your reducing program and you won't have to wait for any "secret ingredients" to slim down.

You can start your diet, Russian style, today.

11

Thirty-Five Ways to Be a Good Loser

1. CHOOSE A DIET YOU CAN LIVE WITH. Follow a definite, well-balanced diet plan, but one that allows for substitutions to suit your taste and way of life. Make it pleasant to stay on by planning it around foods that you enjoy eating, that are easy to prepare and comfortably within your budget.

2. TAKE A DRINK. Drink up first so you'll eat less later. Have an appetite curber in the form of a nonalcoholic and noncaloric drink half an hour before dinner. A cup of consommé, coffee, tea, bouillon, or a tall glass of water or other no-cal beverage will take the edge off your appetite and keep you from overeating.

3. OUTWIT YOUR GULLET. Eat bulky, raw foods that demand vigorous chewing and are filling. Munch a solid wedge of lettuce or raw cabbage between meals or just before meals. A wedge takes longer to eat than a cut-up salad and seems more filling. And all that energetic chomping is good for the teeth and provides exercise that helps firm and tighten a sagging jawline, a slack throat, and a double chin.

4. TAKE A BREATHER. If you're a shallow breather (most of us are), try practicing deep breathing until you do it automatically. Any exercise that makes you breathe deeply is especially good. An authority on diet and exercise, Manya Kahn, says, "Deep breathing flushes the body with oxygen, activates the breathing muscles, *and helps promote the burning of stored, excess fat.*" (My italics.)

5. HASTE MAKES WAIST. Obese people tend to wolf down their food so fast that their appestat doesn't have

time to register "Full!" So they keep right on eating and eating and getting fatter and fatter. If you're guilty of nonstop eating, put a place card beside your plate with these words from Burton's famous *Anatomy of Melancholy* written on it: *"Give food the mouth treatment and you'll be full in half the time."*

6. MEASURE YOUR PROGRESS. Once a week take a tape measure and see how much you've lost in inches. For accuracy, place the tape measure in exactly the same spots each week—the thickest part of your hips, thighs and upper arm (*not* the thinnest!), the bulgiest bulge of your midriff and derrière, etc. An inches-off record can bolster your morale when the scales get stuck in one place (see below). And see the back of the book for charts to record your progress.

7. DON'T WEIGH EVERY DAY. A one-pound variation from day to day can either discourage you or make you overconfident, depending on whether it's up or down. A shift in the fluid balance can cause a temporary increase in weight while you're still losing in inches, so don't let it discourage you. Weigh only once a week, preferably at the same time and wearing the same amount of clothing—or none at all.

8. SET A REALISTIC GOAL FOR YOURSELF. Don't try to lose too much too fast. A steady weight loss of one or two pounds a week has a better chance of being permanent than a fast one. It gives your skin and muscles time to adjust to the loss, prevents a haggard look, and keeps you looking and feeling your best.

9. KEEP A WEIGHT DIARY. Write down how much you weigh when you start your diet and how much you lose each week until you reach your goal. A written record of your weekly weight loss can encourage you to keep on going when you hit a stubborn weight plateau. And it might keep you from cheating, too!

10. DON'T EAT WHEN YOU'RE TIRED AND TENSE. Take time to relax first. Relaxation aids in the digestion and absorption of food, a vital factor in preventing the "hidden hunger" that results in overeating.

11. REACH FOR THE CEILING, NOT FOR A SWEET. S-T-R-E-T-C-H your arms, neck, and torso as high as they will go, then relax in a rag-doll flop. Relieves tension and lessens the frustrations that make you crave candy and other "reward" foods of childhood.

12. BE A GOOD SPORT. Swim, golf, play tennis, bicycle, dance, jog, or jump a real or an imaginary rope. Remember, any activity that makes you breathe hard helps burn stored fat, and consumes some of the excess calories that make fat. An hour of active swimming consumes 670 calories, and regular sessions of it will tighten your muscles and reduce you in inches if not in pounds. So will other vigorous sports and exercises, but in varying degrees.

13. TAKE A WALK. Walking is an exercise that requires only two built-in pieces of equipment—your feet. (Shoes are optional.) Do walk every day, whenever and wherever you can, and make them brisk walks. Walk up and down stairs instead of taking the elevator or escalator. If you can't walk all the way to work or to the market, park your car halfway to your destination and finish the trip on foot.

14. DON'T SLOUCH. Stand tall, tuck in your derrière and tighten those stomach muscles that slouching had made weak and lazy. A good posture promotes better muscle tone and makes you look slimmer.

15. DO EXERCISE EVERY DAY. A combination of diet and exercise will reduce you faster than either one can do alone. As little as 5 to 15 minutes of well-chosen exercises done consistently can firm your contours, flatten your bulges, and help *prevent* a weight gain.

16. BE A SLIM GOURMET. Martin Lederman, the formerly fat diet dropout who became a Slim Gourmet, found that by concentrating on the taste and flavor of each bite of food, and savoring each sip of wine instead of gulping it, he was enjoying his meals more, but was satisfied with less. "If we do not consciously enjoy the first bite," he says, "we eat another and another, and keep on until we're stuffed."

17. TAKE TIME TO TALK. Good conversation takes your mind off food and slows down eating. The Plump Glutton shovels his food in rapidly and silently, seldom lifting his eyes from his plate until he's finished. The Slim Gourmet pauses between bites to talk, to listen, to appreciate the conversation and his surroundings. Actress Paula Prentiss is a Slim Gourmet, who says, "I nibble—and I nibble slowly. Besides, I let myself get so hung-up on conversation that I forget to eat."

18. SERVE YOURSELF SOME SOUL FOOD. Not the kind

you think—most of it's too fattening. But "hyacinths to feed thy soul" are not. Fresh flowers on the table are soul food. (Even a TV tray has room for a single flower in a bud vase.) So is anything else that's lovely to listen to or gaze upon. Soft background music (a Mozart quartet). The glow of candlelight. A table moved near a window with a view of the sunset—or the moon. Add new dimensions to your sense of beauty, taste, sight, and smell to make your meals more enjoyable and less fattening.

19. HABIT PANGS OR HUNGER PANGS? It's habit pangs that you get at dessert time. Eating is governed by habit—and you can change your habits. Listen to your hunger pangs, but discipline your habit pangs and break the dessert habit. Or exchange it for a better one. Like the fresh-fruit habit.

20. SCUTTLE YOUR ALIBIS. Stop blaming heredity ("Fat runs in the family!"), your fat cells and overworked glands. Your salivary glands are the ones that are working overtime. And when you say "Everything I eat turns to fat," it's a pretty safe bet that you're eating too much food that's too high in carbohydrates.

21. MAJOR IN MNEMONICS. Take a tip from Mnemosyne, the goddess of memory, and brush up on yours. Memorize the foods you should eat to slim down and those that put weight on you (pages 192-3)—and don't forget which is which!

22. LIVE OFF THE LEAN OF THE LAND. Trim all visible fat from meat and remove the skin from poultry. Chill casseroles, stews and soups in the refrigerator, skim off the excess fat and reheat. If you use butter at all, use it very sparingly. You'll use less if it's softened or whipped, as it spreads better than hard butter and a little goes a long way. And do use low-fat or powdered skim milk and buttermilk instead of whole milk, which is twice as fattening.

23. DO EAT BREAKFAST EVERY DAY. This is included just as a reminder. The reasons have already been given.

24. FILL YOUR PLATE. Yes, I know you've been told *not* to fill it, but a half-empty plate makes most dieters feel so deprived that they end up raiding the refrigerator later. Keep your eyes from telling your stomach it's being starved by using a smaller plate for smaller portions. Then fill up any empty spaces on it with garnishes of watercress, parsley, carrot curls, cucumber slices, radish roses, or any

of the eat-all-you-want vegetables that are filling and non-fattening.

25. SAVE SOME FOR LATER. It's good psychology to *fill* your plate (with protein and low-carbohydrate food, of course), but you don't have to *clean* it. Remember about dividing meals into snacks? Any of these saved from breakfast, lunch or dinner would be good for a between-meal or bedtime snack: a hard-boiled egg, some of the garnishes from your plate or other "finger salads," a slice of meat, chicken or turkey, a piece of cheese or fruit, or part of your milk allowance for the day.

26. USE SALT SPARINGLY. Find new ways of seasoning with herbs. Try kelp granules for a tangy and unique flavor. Kelp, a rich source of iodine and other minerals from the sea, is available in health-food stores in several different forms. And it has two valuable reducing advant-ages: The regular use of kelp helps prevent fluid retention and steps up the metabolism.

27. SWEAR OFF SUGAR. Every extra lump makes you lumpier. And sugar in several cups of coffee or tea a day can add up to a lot of lumps—and lumpiness! Learn to do without it and you'll soon discover subtle and delightful flavors in both tea and coffee that are disguised by heavy sweetening.

28. BE A PIN-UP. Pin a snapshot taken at your fattest above your mirror. Paste the fattest one of all (maybe a rear view of yourself?) on the refrigerator door.

29. REWARD YOURSELF. After each five-pound weight loss, or after you've resisted some practically irresistible temptation, you deserve a reward. (See the Resist-and-Reward Chart in the back of the book.) It can be any-thing you want to buy yourself—as long as it's nonfatten-ing.

30. MAKE A FOOL-YOURSELF DESSERT. When you're absolutely perishing for a dessert topped with huge mounds of whipped cream, go ahead and have it. Pow-dered skim milk whips beautifully and looks and tastes sinfully rich, but isn't. Sweeten it with a little vanilla or honey and pile it on fresh berries, sliced peaches or other favorite fruit.

31. TRY THE TEENSY SYSTEM. The Teensy System is Roosevelt Grier's method of satisfying his craving for rich food. Rosey, a former football star turned actor, admits that he used to eat "massive quantities" of the foods he

craved. Like two German chocolate cakes or a triple order of lobster Newburg. The Rams gave him an incentive to curb his appetite when they set his weight limit at 287 pounds. Beyond that, a $100 fine was to be paid for each pound that he gained.

"I soon discovered," says Rosey, "that by permitting myself teensies—that is, tiny portions—of these cravings, I could satisfy my mind without expanding my body. I mean, you just don't bring the mind to its knees."

And if a man who once ate two whole chocolate cakes at a sitting can be satisfied with teensies when he makes up his mind to do it, so can you.

32. SUPPLEMENT YOUR DIET. Don't lose your vitality while you're shedding weight. Take a good vitamin-mineral supplement to boost your energy and insure an adequate intake of essential nutrients without adding calories.

33. LIQUIDATE YOUR WEIGHT. Remember the benefits of a day or two of a liquid diet or a modified fast? It's worth trying for one day a week, or for a day or two a month. Even an occasional liquid meal does a lot for some dieters. Let your health and the amount of weight you need to lose be your guide.

34. POSE IN THE NUDE. A doctor and a psychologist suggest that fatties pose naked each day before a full-length mirror and look at themselves from all angles for several minutes. Dr. Daniel Cappon (University of Toronto) and Dr. Robin Banks (University of Waterloo) found that it helped their patients lose weight, but didn't say whether it was from vanity-motivation or disgust-motivation.

35. DELIVER US FROM THESE. In his clever verse, *A Fat Man's Prayer*, the actor Victor Buono lightens his weight problem with a sense of humor. Here are a few condensed lines from his "prayer," which is good advice for all fat persons to follow:

"Lord, grant me strength that I may not fall
Into the clutches of cholesterol . . .
At poly-unsaturates I'll never mutter,
For the Road to Hell is paved with butter;
And cream is cursed and cake is awful
And Satan is hiding in every waffle . . .
Beelzebub is a chocolate drop,
And Lucifer is a lollypop . . .

Teach me the evils of Hollandaise,
Of pasta à la Milanese,
And crisp-fried chicken from the South . . .
LORD, IF YOU LOVE ME, SHUT MY MOUTH!"

(With my apologies to Mr. Buono for the few liberties taken in condensing it to fit in here.)

12

How to Kick the Flab Habit

Do you have hypokinesis?

No, it isn't contagious. And it isn't necessary to call in a hypokinesis specialist, even if there were any, which there aren't. Although complications develop from it if it isn't corrected, the remedy is a simple one that you can apply yourself.

You begin the cure by kicking the flab habit.

Hypokinesis is the scientific name for an old condition that afflicts the fat, flabby, and physically inactive person.

It's a condition that creates its own destructive circle: If you're a victim of hypokinesis you've been avoiding physical activity, evading exercise and shunning the sports you used to enjoy. And the more you avoid them the worse you get. Weak, flabby muscles grow weaker and flabbier, and a continuing lack of exercise results in a steady physical decline.

First, the flabby arms, jowls, abdomen and seat, an increasing muscular weakness and chronic fatigue, all of which make you look and feel older than you are.

That's bad enough, but it isn't all. The flabbiness doesn't stop there. Unless it is checked it will go on to affect the blood vessels, the respiratory system, the muscles of the heart and other vital organs.

"The wise, for cure, on exercise depend," wrote poet John Dryden more than two and a half centuries ago.

Exercise, not diet, is the cure for flabbiness. And if you start in time you won't need a cure. Exercise will *prevent* it, and keep you firm, trim, and flexible as long as you keep it up.

"There is strong authoritative support," says the President's Council on Physical Fitness, "for the concept that *regular exercise can prevent degenerative diseases and slow down the physical deterioration that accompanies aging."* (My italics.)

More than half of your body is comprised of muscle. When you gain weight, fat settles around them. Weakened by disuse and the burden of excess fat, muscles stretch and sag. You can lose weight by dieting, but muscles that have been stretched will continue to sag unless you strengthen and firm them with exercise.

What Exercise Can and Cannot Do

Can exercise reduce you?

To some extent, yes. But losing weight by exercise alone is a slow process. You've probably heard that you'd have to walk 30 hours, more or less, to lose a pound of fat. (It depends upon how briskly you walk and how fast you burn calories. Since it varies with the individual, the experts don't agree on this. Some say that walking burns 115 calories an hour, others claim up to 300.)

But before you rule out exercise as a reducing aid, listen to what Dr. Joseph C. Molnar said about it.

"It takes a lot of exercise," he wrote, "to use up an ounce of fat. But let's look at it this way: If it's only enough exercise to use up an ounce of fat a day, that's still 22 pounds in a year. Losing (or not gaining) this amount in a year is a big achievement. Except in the rarest cases, 22 pounds in a year is the difference between normal weight and great corpulence. An ounce a day!"

A study reported in *Nutrition Reviews* (4:69) indicates that exercise does much more to help you lose weight than merely improve the balance of your calorie intake and energy output. Exercise is now believed to provoke a more rapid turnover of the free fatty acids. If that doesn't mean anything to you, this part of it will:

It influences your overall metabolism. And if you've done your homework you know that a stepped-up metabolism burns fat faster.

Exercise can tighten sagging contours, tone and firm your muscles, tendons, and connective tissue and reshape your proportions. And since fat tends to accumulate on the least-exercised muscles, exercise can prevent future fat formation.

Exercise can pare bulges of fat from your bones, but it can't alter your bone structure. If you have wide hip bones, exercise can slim them by giving them leaner lines and smooth, trim contours, but it can't narrow them.

Only exercise can keep our bodies from eventually changing into a grotesque shape, according to a California doctor.

"The shape of the human body is gradually changing," warns Dr. William S. Leonard of Los Angeles. "If we don't do something about it, one of these days the human being will have a big head, small shoulders, a round back, a big, heavy seat and thighs, and tiny, skinny legs."

Does that resemble anyone you know?

"Just look around," continues Dr. Leonard, "and you will notice the tendency toward being pear-shaped even among our youngsters. In the modern society, people do less than one-fourth the walking they should."

Kicking the flab habit will prevent hypokinesis and keep you from getting pear-shaped. And the best way to break the habit is to do something that gets you off your seat and on your feet. Almost any exercise, sport or diversion that keeps you moving instead of sitting will do it.

Dr. Leonard recommends that Americans go back to walking, and so does every authority on weight control and physical fitness.

Dr. Frederick Stare, who in his late fifties keeps as lean and lithe as he did in his twenties, says, "I simply have to burn energy or my weight goes up, so I walk. And when I walk, I walk like hell—with real gusto."

The girls are given an incentive to walk by Dr. Morton Walker, a Stamford, Connecticut podiatrist, who says this about it:

"Daily walks increase sex appeal when flabby thighs firm up and calf muscles develop shapely and well-defined curves."

Walk, then, to kick the flab habit, to get in shape, keep in shape—and to develop sex appeal. (I mean *more* sex appeal, of course!) Dance, play tennis, ride a bicycle or swim for the same reasons.

You don't know how to dance, can't play tennis, don't own a bicycle, and never learned to swim?

All right. You *do* know how to walk. So walk as often as you can. Consistently. And briskly. And you can do the familiar bicycle exercise without a bicycle. Or jump an imaginary rope. You don't have to own one—just imagine it. Or jog. No special skills or equipment needed for these.

Jog or run in place indoors. Or jog outdoors covering actual ground. But be sure it's on the ground. *Never* run or jog on the sidewalk or pavement—the hard, jolting impact can be injurious.

Don't start out as though you're training for the Olympics. *But do demand more of your store of physical energy.*

"What store of energy?" you ask.

If yours is in short supply, exercise can help restore it.

The famous Dr. Paul Dudley White recommends exercise to revitalize the body, stimulate the circulation, improve the breathing, and strengthen and firm the muscles, including the heart muscles. In his opinion, exercises "that challenge the legs" will do this, and his own favorites are brisk walking and bicycling.

Whatever you choose, it should be something that suits your taste, temperament, age, and physical capacity. But remember that weak, flabby muscles must be conditioned gradually to prevent stiffness and soreness. So walk before you run or jog. And start exercising with warm-ups, not push-ups. Here are some easy ones that you can do before you get out of bed in the morning.

Warm-Ups in Bed

A few minutes of warm-ups while lying in bed can relieve muscular stiffness and tension, redistribute the blood and step up the circulation, increase early-morning mental alertness and muscular flexibility, and give you energy to start the day.

1.

Lie flat on your back, arms extended toward the head of the bed. Stretch slowly but hard 6 times, elongating the body as much as possible. Hold each stretch for a few seconds, then relax briefly before starting the next one.

2.

With arms beside the body, hands palms down on the bed (for support, if necessary!) and legs together with knees slightly bent, arch back 3 times, lifting it clear of the bed each time.

3.

Do 3 sit-ups touching the toes. Gradually work up to a total of 10. (When you "graduate" from this, do 10 sit-ups touching forehead to knees.)

4.

Tense all leg muscles hard and relax. Repeat for a total of 12 times.

5.

Do 3 leg-lifts. With legs together, raise them slowly from the bed to point toward the ceiling. Hold a moment before lowering them slowly to the bed. As your abdominal muscles strengthen, gradually work up to 10 leg-lifts.

6.

Draw in the abdomen hard—harder! Hold until the muscles start to quiver, then let it out. Place hands on abdomen and push vigorously while resisting by tensing abdominal muscles. Draw in. Hold. Relax. Push. Tense. Hold. Relax. Repeat 10 times.

7.

Drop chin to chest. Lift chin and slowly stretch neck up and out to the right, lowering head down toward the right shoulder until you feel the pull on the neck muscles. Relax. Repeat on left side. Five times on each side.

8.

Raise bent knees over your head and touch ears with knees 4 times. (Come, now—that's not so difficult! But if you think it is, start out by touching knees to chest until you limber up.)

Exercise will keep you from being the girl with her limber lost. Or the middle-aged man or woman. Or the senior citizen.

No matter how busy you are, whether you're a housewife or a business executive, you can find opportunities to stretch, bend, and twist as you go about your work.

Exercises to Watch TV By

Like to watch TV? Well, don't just *sit* there. Stretch. Bend. Twist. And kick. Firm the muscles of the diaphragm, abdomen, waist, hips, thighs, and legs while you're watching. Keep your blood circulating instead of stagnating.

1. Get up and jog in place during the minute and a half commercial.

2. Kick off your shoes and walk on tiptoe when you go to get a drink of water.

3. Walk back from the kitchen like a drum majorette, lifting knees waist-high with each step.

4. Plant both feet firmly on the carpet, digging in hard as though to push them through the floor, until you feel the pull on every muscle in your body. Hold for a count of 10. Relax. Ready to sit down and watch the picture? All right. But don't slump back on your spine.

5. Sit tall, stretching upward as far as you can. Stretch your neck up out of your shoulders. Lift your rib cage high, feel your body pulling up from your hips. With your back straight, bend from side to side, good, deep bends, as near the floor as you can go without toppling off your chair. Six bends on each side.

6. Sit with back braced against your chair, hands gripping the sides. With legs together, bend knees and slowly bring them up to the chest. Repeat 6 times.

7. With back still braced against the chair and hands gripping the sides, raise legs in front of you and do the scissors kick, kicking the right leg across the left at hip level, then the left leg across the right. Rapidly. Twenty times, or until your legs get tired—whichever comes first.

8. Plant your feet firmly on the floor. Lean forward to

grasp your legs as far down as you can—at the ankle if you can make it that far. Hold on tightly, against resistance, and pull straight up as though to lift the legs from the floor. Lift hard enough and resist enough and you'll feel the pull in your derrière, arms and back.

Who said exercise was hard? Here you've already had sixteen limbering, firming and toning routines without getting out of bed or off your chair—except during the TV commercials!

"But I need more than that," some of you tell me. "My weight's all right now, but my proportions aren't. How can I get rid of a bulgy abdomen and thick, lumpy hips and thighs?"

If you're thick and tired of it, here are some special exercises for problem spots.

Waist, Hip, Derrière and Thigh Trimmers

1. *The Hip Spanker.* When your hips spank on the floor, something has to give—and it won't be the floor! Lie on back, bend your legs, bringing knees up toward your waist.

Swing knees from left to right, rolling rapidly from one side to the other until your thighs spank the floor hard on each side. Start with 8 hip spanks on each side and work up to 16. (Or 26 if they're *really* thick.)

2. *The Fanny Walk.* This is one of the 10 Best Exercises on almost everybody's list. Better wear heavy-duty jeans or reinforced slacks for it.

Sit flat on the floor with legs out straight and arms folded across your chest. Wiggle forward across the room, shifting the weight from side to side with each "step" you take. Let your knees bend slightly as you shift weight and "step" forward. Take 10 forward steps and 10 backward, gradually working up to a total of 5 complete forward and backward walks of 10 steps each.

3. *The Side Scissors-Kick.* This is a little harder than the one you did while watching TV, and it's also more effective.

Lie on your right side on the floor, head pillowed on arm, legs straight down, one resting on top of the other. Raise both legs slightly from floor and shuttle into the scissors kick for a count of 10. Change sides and repeat 10 times.

4. *The Leg Orbit.* Same position as above. Raise top leg, keeping knee straight, and swing leg up and around in wide circles, 6 slow, wide circles in one direction, 6 in another. Change sides and circle with the opposite leg.

5. *Abdomen, Hips and Fanny Flattener.* Get down on your hands and knees and bring your right knee forward as close to your nose as possible. Raise your head as you stretch the leg back and up, lifting leg as high as you can. Repeat with left knee and leg (same nose!), 10 times to each side, gradually working up to 20 times to each side.

6. *The Saddlebags Slimmers.* Bonnie Prudden calls them "saddlebags" and Jack LaLanne's name for them is "the jodhpur bulge." They're the bulges on the outside of the upper thigh, the pads of fat that both overweight and underweight persons often have. Because "saddlebags" are both prominent and hard to lose, here are three exercises for them. The first is recommended by Mrs. Prudden, the second by Jack LaLanne, and the third is one used by Miss Marjorie Craig in her famous exercise lessons at Elizabeth Arden's in New York.

I.

Get down on your hands and knees. Keeping the knee bent, raise the right leg on the side to hip level, if you can. Stretch the leg straight out to the side and holding it at hip level bend the knee again. Without lowering leg, straighten it and swing it straight back. Hold briefly before lowering it to the floor in the starting position. Repeat with left leg. Start with 2 to each side; work up to 8 or 10. (For obvious reasons Mrs. Prudden sometimes calls this exercise "The Hydrant.")

II.

Lie on right side, turning so your abdomen almost faces the floor. Lift your left leg up and back as high as you can. Feel the pull in your hip and bustle muscles? Then lower leg slowly to the floor. Roll over on left side and repeat with the right leg. Five times with each leg to start. Work up to 10 or 15 times with each leg.

III.

This one is similar to number II, but a little more difficult. Lie on your side with head pillowed on outstretched underneath arm. Raise your top leg up. Raise your bottom leg up to meet it. Hold legs together in midair. Lower your bottom leg slowly to the floor. Follow it slowly with your top leg. Do exercise 5 times. Roll over and repeat on opposite side. Work up to 10 or 12 times on each side.

Hips and Waist Whittlers

7. *The Jackknife*. Lie on back with arms outstretched in front of you. Sit up slowly, and at the same time bring your legs up, keeping legs and back straight as you balance on your derrière so your body forms a half-open jackknife (or the letter V). Start with 4, work up to 10.

8. *The Twist and Toe-Touch*. Stand with feet 18 to 24 inches apart. Bend from waist, as far back and as far to the right as you can. Circle body around, lean forward from waist and twist torso to touch toes of left foot with right hand.

Repeat backward bend, circle and twist on left side, touching toes of right foot with left hand. Six times on each side to start. Work up to a total of 20.

Arm and Bosom Firmers

9. *The Handcuff Stretch*. Stand with feet apart, hands clasped firmly behind you. Bend forward from hips, keeping back straight. With fingers tightly locked, stretch arms up over back toward shoulder level as high as possible. Repeat 10 times.

10. *Hand-to-Hand Combat*. Clasp hands in front of you at shoulder level, fingers tightly interlocked and forearms horizontal. Push palms hard against each other until you feel the pull on underarms and pectoral muscles. Ten times to start, three times a day, gradually working up to 20 or 30.

11. *Dry Swimming: The Breast Stroke*. Swimming is a great way to slim down or build up the parts of your body

that need it. It strengthens the muscles, "challenges the legs," fights flab in unwanted places, reduces or develops you as needed, and streamlines your proportions.

If you live near the water or have access to a swimming pool, do swim regularly. If not, practice the strokes on dry land.

The breast stroke firms the arms and firms and lifts the breasts by developing the pectoral muscles that hold them up. Here's how you can do it without going near the water:

Sit on the floor with legs outstretched in front of you, rib cage lifted, back straight and palms together in front of chest. Keep palms together and shoot arms straight out in front of you. Turn palms outward and thrust arms in an arc behind you as far as possible. Then bend elbows and bring arms forward to starting position in front of chest again. Movements should flow into each other rhythmically but vigorously, so you can feel the pull in chest, arms, shoulders and back.

12. *Chin and Neck "Sit-ups."* To undouble the chin, firm the neck and tighten a sagging jawline.

Lie on your back across the side of a bed with head and neck hanging down over the edge. Keep your head upside down a minute until you feel the flow of circulation in your face. Then keeping the shoulders flat on the bed, slowly raise your head and neck to a "sitting" position and rotate head from side to side before lowering chin to chest. Lift chin from chest and slowly lower head and neck down over the edge of the bed again. Start with 5. Work up to 12 or 15, but do it gradually to keep from getting a stiff neck.

The ideal way to lose weight, get rid of flab and bulges in problem spots and prevent an allover sag of muscles can be summed up in four words:

Eat less—exercise more!

As the years pass, keeping slim becomes a battle to the death (literally!) between two groups of opposing forces . . .

Appetite, Inactivity, and Overweight
versus
You, Diet, and Exercise.

Who's going to win?

13

Obesity and Your Sex Life

Does excessive overweight result in a loss of sex drive and capacity?

Hundreds of case histories of obese men and women give evidence that it does.

In clinical experience with obese patients, Dr. Frank S. Caprio, noted for his research and writings on the sexually adequate male, has seen many examples of the relation between obesity and sexual inadequacy.

"Some men suffer from what is called 'nutritive libido,'" says Dr. Caprio, "—a food drive comparable to the sex drive except that they get more pleasure out of frequent and excessive eating than their physical relations with their wives."

The same is true of the grossly overweight woman who finds more satisfaction in food than she does in the love of her husband. How can such a woman—or man—with a nutritive libido, who prefers food to love, be a total partner in love and marriage?

Instead of finding normal outlets for their tensions and frustrations, they eat to relieve them. When they feel angry or rejected they turn to food for comfort, and unless the habit can be broken it becomes a permanent way of life.

Ultimately they have neither the energy nor the desire for total involvement in anything. They accept a loss of sexual interest as normal and settle for levels of desire and potency far below what they should have.

I glanced at the appointment book on my desk and saw that my next interview was marked *Urgent*. When Roscoe Hale walked in, one look at him revealed that "urgent"

was an understatement. "Critical" was a better description
of his problem.

He eased his enormous bulk into a chair and started to
cross his legs before remembering that the size of his
potbelly made it physically impossible for him to do so. "I
have a problem," he began. "Can you help me?"

"I've helped others in the same condition," I assured
him. "I can help you, too, if you'll cooperate."

His three chins bobbled up and down as he nodded.
"Well, sure. But you'll have to get my wife's cooperation.
She's the problem."

"You mean your *wife* has a worse weight problem than
yours?" I asked.

"Oh, no. She's slim. Always has been. Weight has nothing to do with our problem. The trouble is—I think she's
going to leave me."

I looked at the anxious eyes, the fat, bloated face and
mounds of sagging flesh spilling over the sides of the chair
and wondered how he could possibly have convinced himself that weight had nothing to do with his marital problems.
Before he could be helped, I thought, he had to be
motivated to look at himself and the situation realistically.

Aloud I said, "Have you asked your wife why she wants
to leave you?"

"It wouldn't do any good. She'd just blame me. And it
isn't my fault. I've given her everything she wants."

"Everything?" I asked, but he was too immersed in
self-pity to notice the inference.

"Ask anybody who knows us. They'll tell you—I'm a
good provider!"

"Mr. Hale, I'm a nutritionist, not a marriage counselor,
but I know that a woman expects her husband to be more
than just a 'good provider.' Why don't you see a—"

"Look," he interrupted, "I've read about lots of failing
marriages you've helped. And I know a couple you kept
from breaking up. Why won't you help my wife?"

It isn't easy to help a man who won't admit that he
needs it, but I said, "All right. I'll do what I can. But first,
we have to look at the problem objectively and decide
whose it *really* is. And if we're going to resolve it you'll
have to level with me. Why does your wife want to leave
you?"

He hesitated and cleared his throat nervously before

answering. "She—says I'm not sexy anymore—that I'm just a fat slob!"

"Psychiatrists who deal with the emotional problems of obesity say that it's hard to be fat and sexy," I said. "You have to realize that obesity is a disease, and that your sexual capacity is directly related to your physical and emotional health."

He lowered his gaze to the floor and mumbled, "I didn't say anything about sexual capacity."

"Isn't that the real problem?" I asked. "First, an excessive gain in weight, then a loss of interest in sex followed by a decrease in capacity?"

He didn't answer, so I continued. "When did you begin to substitute food for sex?"

For a moment I thought he hadn't heard me, and when he began to speak the words came slowly and painfully.

"I think ... it began at a club dance about two years ago. I was always a good dancer ... lots of fat men are, you know."

"Yes, I know."

"Lois—that's my wife—loves to dance. Besides, I wasn't quite so fat two years ago. But she was already after me to go on a diet. Said she couldn't stand to see me going to pot." He patted his stomach. "And that night in the middle of a dance she told me it was impossible to dance with me—my stomach got in the way. Then she walked off the floor and left me standing there alone."

"What did you do?"

"Headed straight for the buffet where the other fat guys gathered, and stuffed myself the rest of the evening."

My secretary came into the office with a pot of herb tea and poured each of us a cup. He looked for sugar, didn't see it, and settled for several spoons of honey. "That's the way it is now every time we go to the club. Lois dances with all the slim, good-looking guys—and I eat."

"What about your home life? Has that changed for the worse?"

"My home life?" He gulped the rest of his tea and stared intently into the empty cup, scraping the honey from the bottom and licking the spoon like a greedy child. "It started falling apart about the same time. My ... my stomach got in the way in the bedroom, too."

He was still licking honey from the spoon the way a

first-grader licks an ice cream cone, wholly absorbed in its flavor.

Watching him, I remembered what psychiatrist Dr. Theodore Rubin had said: that grossly overweight patients have a "complete emotional investment in food" which leaves them little or no emotional energy for love.

According to the psychiatrist, *"Obese people almost always have sexual problems."*

Years of treating the problems of obesity have convinced Dr. Rubin that compulsive eating is a form of displaced sexualization, and he says, "To fat people, there is much sensuality in their eating and much dissipation of sexual feelings ... which is very destructive to closeness and good sexual relations."

Roscoe Hale's next remark substantiated Dr. Rubin's statement. "It got so the only pleasure I had at home was a midnight raid on the refrigerator after my wife was asleep. I look forward to that all evening. You might not believe it to look at me, but it's my only big meal of the day."

"I believe you. A lot of overweight persons do most of their eating between meals and during the late evening hours. But I'd like to know what motivates you. Why would you rather eat alone than with others—even your wife?"

His face flushed with embarrassment, but his answer was honest. "It's obvious, isn't it? One look at me and everybody thinks I'm a glutton."

"If you want to prove them wrong," I said, "there's a better way of doing it than starving yourself of essential nutrients at meals and eating a lot of fattening food when nobody's looking. It's a familiar pattern among the obese. Some of them are ashamed of their ravenous appetites, so to keep it a secret they eat very little in company but stuff themselves in solitude. Then there are the wishful thinkers who kid themselves into thinking that what they eat in private doesn't show in public. And one of your problems—the midnight raids on the refrigerator—is often a problem of sexual frustration."

"I've wondered about that," he admitted. "I know that my worst food binges began after my wife humiliated me in public. Now I can't control them. They seem all mixed up with hunger, sexual frustration, a loss of confidence—and wanting to punish her for rejecting me."

"It's not uncommon for excessively overweight men and women to use their fatness as a security blanket—and as a surreptitious weapon. Many of those I've treated have told me that they decided to diet because their mates found obesity sexually repulsive, and they wanted to regain the love and admiration they had lost."

"Like my wife and me," said Roscoe.

"But let them get angry with the one they love and some will use it as an excuse to stop dieting, start stuffing themselves, and get fatter than ever as a means of 'getting even.' These are the emotionally immature diet dropouts who need help in resolving their hang-ups before they can lose weight successfully."

"That's my wife for you." He couldn't resist bringing her into it again. "Emotionally immature."

"Look, why don't we stick to the point?" I asked. "We're talking of the sexual problems of obesity, and you say she's slim."

But he was so eager to prove his point that mine failed to register. "I used to think that if we had children Lois would grow up emotionally. If that had happened, our marriage wouldn't be on the rocks now. That was before I knew she couldn't have any."

"Are you sure it's your wife who can't?"

"Well, we've been married twelve years—and both of us wanted children."

"Did you know that overeating and obesity are major factors in sterility?" I asked.

"You mean you think that I. . . ."

"It could be either of you. There's no way of knowing without a test. But many hospital experiments, including the extensive studies at the sterility clinic of Cedars of Lebanon Hospital in Los Angeles, have shown that a physical condition such as yours can and often does result in sterility. Maybe yours hasn't. But why not prevent it by getting your weight back to normal and increasing your sexual vigor and capacity at the same time?"

His eyes were focused on the picture of my daughter on my desk, and he spoke slowly, without looking at me. "I've been kidding myself all along—and you knew it. All this time I've been projecting, blaming my wife because I couldn't bear to admit that I was fat, repulsive, and losing interest in sex. Well, now I've admitted it. What do I do now?"

"You go on a diet designed to take weight off and build up your health—a diet that supplies all the essential nutrients your body must have to burn fat efficiently. Fat burns faster and more efficiently on a high-protein diet, so you'll feature protein in all your meals."

"Sounds easy so far. Is that all there is to it?"

"Not quite. I'd like to talk to your wife about your diet and make some suggestions to her for your special problems."

"Well, sure, if you want to," he agreed, but his voice was uncertain. "Just don't forget—she's threatened to leave me. Says I'm not the man she married."

"Don't you think she might change her mind if there's a chance of getting that man back?" I asked.

"You know something?" A glimmer of hope began chasing the gloom from his face. "She just might do it—if *you* put it to her that way."

That's exactly the way I put it to Mrs. Hale, and it worked.

"Of course I used to love him," she said. "I suppose I still do, in a way. I simply can't stand the big fat slob he's become. But if he's willing to go on a diet and stay on it I'll do what I can to help."

"Your husband's been going on these food binges instead of eating with you because he feels frustrated and rejected. To restore his ego and build up his confidence, let's work out a romantic diet for him."

"A *what?*"

"The basic diet will be what I always recommend: eggs, lean meat, fish, poultry, cottage cheese, skim milk, 2 leafy green salads a day, all the vegetables he can eat chosen from an eat-all-you-want list I'll give you, plus ½ grapefruit or other citrus fruit and one other low-carbohydrate fruit a day. It's the way you'll serve it that will make it romantic."

Roscoe's Romantic Diet

Mrs. Hale cooperated by setting the scene for romance. Dinner by candlelight, flowers on the table, a background of soft music, and a glass of chilled, very dry wine to set the mood (and relax the tensions and aid digestion).

"We want to break his pattern of solitary eating by getting his mind off refrigerator raids and on you," I told her, "so wear something soft, clinging and sexy. I know it sounds corny, but I think what he needs to get him started is a little special attention from a charming, feminine woman who can build up his confidence and make him feel like a man again."

Here is the low-carbohydrate, high-vitality menu we planned for the first dinner of Roscoe's Romantic Diet.

> Bouillon with sliced mushrooms and celery
> Broiled lobster
> Fresh asparagus
> Leafy green salad with safflower oil and vinegar
> Small wedge of cheese
> Black coffee

The next day Mrs. Hale called to tell me, "Roscoe was so pleased with the relaxed atmosphere and the fact that I'd prepared everything especially for him that he didn't even miss bread, potatoes and dessert. There were no refrigerator raids last night! And you should have seen how eagerly he drank his bedtime snack of skim milk and lecithin when I told him it was a fat-emulsifier and a virility booster!"

I had recommended a tablespoon of lecithin granules dissolved in half a glass of skim milk or tomato juice twice a day for Roscoe. In my opinion, it's essential for every man who wants to retain or regain his sexual vigor, and for every obese man or woman, to aid the body's utilization of fats and help the cells burn fat.

Here are other food supplements that helped Roscoe reduce and regain his vitality at the same time:

A *multi-vitamin-mineral supplement*. It takes all the essential nutrients to aid the fat-burning process—and the high-carbohydrate foods that had put weight on Roscoe had short-changed him nutritionally. The fastest way to make up deficiencies is by adding concentrated supplements to a balanced diet. (A formula that I recommend very highly is available under the name of Nutri-Time.)

B-Complex. A deficiency of any of the B-vitamins causes a slowdown in energy production. Since it's only when energy is produced that fat is lost, it's a good idea to stock up on B-vitamins if you're trying to lose weight. And make it the whole B-complex instead of single B-vitamins or you might lose out on the ones you need the most. If you're deficient in just one of them, pantothenic acid, fats burn at only half their normal rate. And a deficiency of B-1 (thiamine) can cause a craving for sweets that will pile more pounds on you.

Vitamin E. Fat is utilized twice as fast when vitamin E is added to a diet that's low in it or in protein. Sometimes called the fertility or virility vitamin, it has been highly successful in restoring sexual vigor and capacity, even in cases of impotence.

Formula HOV. You already know the many ways that HOV fights fat and why it's included in Roscoe's Romantic Diet—and I hope in yours, too!

Liver—any kind. At least two times a week, especially in Roscoe's case, for its B-12, choline, iron and zinc content. Without choline and another B-vitamin, B-6, protein is changed to fat instead of being the fat fighter it normally is. And it's a matter of record that a deficiency of B-12 (often noted among vegetarians) leads to decreased sexual desire and capacity.

Vitamin C. As we grow older and our hormone production slows down we need larger amounts of vitamin C in our diets, or taken as supplements. This is especially true of men, whose sex glands require it to keep them functioning normally as the years pass.

Some of these items on Roscoe's Romantic Diet don't *sound* romantic, but his wife tells me that the effects of them are.

As of this writing, Roscoe has been on the diet for 5½ months and lost 64 pounds. He and Mrs. Hale were in to see me recently, and he patted his almost-flat stomach proudly.

"Now this doesn't get in the way on the dance floor," he said, and winked, "or anywhere else."

Mrs. Hale took my hand in both of hers and said, "When I think of the shape Roscoe was in, I just don't know how to thank you. You saved our marriage."

"The Romantic Diet did more than that," I said. "It saved Roscoe's life."

If you're fat and fed up with it, why not try a romantic diet of your own?

Getting your weight back to normal can improve your health, enhance your sexuality, and make you the total partner in love and marriage you would like to be.

The person you can be.

14

Slimming Recipes That Satisfy

"Haven't you gained a lot more weight?" I asked Alan Marsden.

It wasn't a tactful question, but Alan was a friend and I was concerned about his health.

He took refuge behind the Fifth Amendment and an uneasy smile. Anyway, an answer wasn't necessary.

All I had to do was look at him.

Less than three months ago Alan's doctor had warned him that he had to lose weight. He was told to start eating as though his life depended on it—because it did!

"What happened to your diet?" I asked.

"Too monotonous. And too expensive for a retired teacher. Besides, I was always hungry on it."

"What you need," I told him, "is a diet that does just the opposite on all three counts."

Good reducing menus should be varied, not monotonous. (The only exceptions are the two or three day mono-diets as an emergency measure when a few pounds have to be shed in a hurry.)

The food doesn't have to be expensive. As I've said, cheaper cuts of meat contain the same high-grade protein as steak, and are usually a lot lower in fat content and calories. The same is true of chicken, turkey, fish and seafood.

And a diet is self-defeating if it leaves you so hungry you can't stay on it.

Monotony. Expense. And hunger.

Some of the reducing tips and recipes that follow helped Alan Marsden beat these three diet-wreckers that threaten all reducers.

They can do the same for you.

How to Diet in Different Languages

Food, like music or a smile, is a universal way of communicating. A language understood by everyone, any place in the world.

Mrs. Graham D. Mattison is an internationally known hostess who lives in New York, Paris, and Cascais in Portugal—when she and her husband aren't traveling in other parts of the world.

Wherever she lives and entertains, Mrs. Mattison's distinguished guests of assorted nationalities have one thing in common. Almost all of them are on some kind of a diet. Her secrets of serving slimming gourmet meals are basic, simple, and easy enough for anyone to follow.

"We never serve very rich food," she says, and plans her menus "so that everyone can eat something to his heart's content" without breaking his diet.

She tells her chefs that sauces must be served in a sauce boat, not on the food. The sauces are often as simple and nonfattening as a purée of celery or mushrooms (easy to make in a blender, thinned with a little milk and seasoned to taste).

"Food is so often dull, routine or too rich," says Mrs. Mattison. She avoids these diet traps—and so can you!—by a sedulous search for original ideas, recipes, and food combinations and by making up new menus and trying them out. With some menus she suggests several different purées in a variety of tastes and colors: cauliflower, carrots, dark green watercress and lighter string beans.

Other favorite purées of hers are sauces and topping made of fresh fruit and berries. Serve a purée of fresh peaches, apricots, or apples with meat or chicken, or make up your own combination of fresh fruits or berries with a contrasting sauce for dessert. (My own favorite is fresh peaches topped with a puréed sauce of raspberries—delicious!) But remember that fruits are high in carbohydrates, so keep the portions small and count both the fruit and the sauce as part of your fruit allowance for the day.

Mrs. Mattison's dinners always include:

Three vegetables, two of them green. (The ones she serves most often are some of those on our eat-all-you-want list.)

A salad, which may be as simple as lettuce hearts, romaine, or a mixed green salad sprinkled with grated egg yolk for a contrast in color and texture.

Cheeses. "Always a dry cheese and a Brie or Camembert," she says.

For nondieters she has a fresh fruit tart or *sablé*. Dieters can enjoy them, too, if they follow her example of eating the fruit but not the crust.

Among the recipes are some of my own favorites, some that I have collected from travels abroad, and two of Mrs. Mattison's French veal recipes on page 150. (Veal is one of the leanest meats, very popular in France, and she serves it frequently, along with *Filets de Sole*.)

A single chapter can't hold all of the recipes that I would like to include. But the selection is still large enough to take the monotony out of meals and add variety to them at no additional cost. To slim you down safely and satisfy your appetite at the same time.

Appetizers—Who Needs Them?

Except for the educated nibble (raw vegetables) and a few slimming snacks of protein, I'd say skip appetizers. The question is, can you educate *your* nibble to resist the rich, fattening ones and reach for those that aren't?

Here are just a few for starters. The first is one that California's famous Golden Door serves to the Beautiful People who go there to reduce and grow more beautiful.

GOLDEN DOOR EDUCATED NIBBLES

Celery stuffed with chopped chicken livers
Raw cauliflower dipped in yogurt
Raw mushrooms stuffed with Cheddar cheese
Cucumber slices
Carrot sticks
Green pepper rings
Cherry or plum tomatoes

EGGPLANT "CAVIAR"

1 large eggplant
1 small onion, finely chopped
1 tomato
Sea salt, pepper, vinegar, oil

Boil or bake eggplant, then peel. If boiled, drain thoroughly; if baked, scoop out insides. Chop eggplant with onion and tomato, adding salt, pepper, vinegar, and oil to taste. Serve cold. Makes 12 hors d'oeuvres servings.

Slimming Protein Snacks

· STUFFED MUSHROOMS

2 cans (6 oz each) mushroom crowns
8 oz skim-milk cottage cheese
2 tbsp minced chives
Dash of hot pepper sauce
⅛ tsp Worcestershire
½ tsp celery salt
½ tsp dry mustard

Drain mushrooms and hollow out stem sides slightly. Mix remaining ingredients and top each crown with some of the mixture. Makes 24.

CHICKEN-LIVER SPREAD

½ lb chicken livers
Water
Sea salt
1 medium onion, minced
½ cup tomato juice
1 hard-cooked egg, finely chopped
2 tbsp minced parsley
2 tsp lemon juice
Pepper to taste

Cover chicken livers with cold water; add ½ tsp salt. Bring to boil and simmer 4 to 5 minutes. Drain and chop fine. Simmer onion in tomato juice 15 minutes. Mix all ingredients. Pack into 1½ cup mold and chill. Unmold and serve with sliced raw zucchini and carrot sticks. Makes about 1½ cups.

ZIPPY CHEESE SPREAD

12 oz pot cheese
½ cup buttermilk
1 tsp seasoned salt
½ tsp seasoned pepper

Combine cheese and buttermilk. Beat until fluffy and well blended. Add seasonings and chill. Makes about 1½ cups.

NIPPY SARDINE SPREAD

1 3¼-to-4-oz can sardines, mashed
¼ cup catsup
½ cup diet cottage cheese
2 tbsp onion, minced
2 tbsp green pepper, finely chopped
¼ tsp red pepper sauce
1 tbsp lemon juice
2 tbsp parsley or watercress, chopped

Combine first 7 ingredients and chill. Garnish with watercress or parsley when ready to serve. Makes 1⅓ cups, plus.

RED SALMON CREAM DIP

½ cup red salmon, flaked
½ cup finely diced cucumber
2 tsp chives, finely cut
1 cup yogurt

Fold salmon, chives and cucumber into yogurt. Chill. Makes 2 cups.

CRAB AND WATER-CHESTNUT DIP

1 6½- to 7-oz can crabmeat, drained and flaked
½ cup (small can) water chestnuts, drained and sliced
1 tbsp soy sauce
3 tbsp low-calorie mayonnaise
2 tbsp freeze-dried frozen, or fresh chives

Mix last 3 ingredients together, then toss with crab and chestnuts. Chill. Makes 1¾ cups.

DIPSY DOODLE DIP

½ cup yogurt
1 cup cottage cheese
¼ cup tomato juice
1 tbsp onion flakes
¼ tsp dry mustard
1 tsp lemon juice
2 tbsp catsup
1 tsp soy sauce

Sieve cottage cheese and fold in yogurt. Blend in onion flakes and mustard. Add soy sauce, catsup, and tomato and lemon juice. Mix thoroughly and chill. Makes 1½ cups.

And, finally, before we stop dipsy doodling with dips, here's a recipe originated by Neil Hulbert, a member of the Board of Directors of the California Beef Council. Not exactly an appetizer, not a spread or dip. Just a real man-pleasing protein snack. (It's a good after-school kid pleaser, too.)

CALIFORNIA BEEF JERKY

1 beef flank steak, well-trimmed
½ cup soy sauce
Garlic salt
Lemon pepper

Cut steak lengthwise with grain into long strips, no more than ¼-inch thick. Toss with soy sauce. Arrange beef strips in single layer on wire rack placed on baking sheet. Sprinkle with garlic salt and lemon pepper. Place second rack over beef and flip over. Remove top rack. Sprinkle again with seasonings. Bake in very slow oven (150 to 175 degrees) overnight, about 10 to 12 hours. Store in covered container. Note: Beef Jerky should not be crisp. If it is, oven temperature is too high.

Thin Soups for Fat People

Thin, clear soups are "comfort" foods. They can soothe an empty stomach without pooching it out. If yours is already pooched, let these thin soups help satisfy and flatten it.

CHICKEN-BROCCOLI BROTH

3 cups boiling water
4 packets flavored instant chicken broth
4 tbsp leftover chicken or turkey, chopped (all white meat)
½ cup broccoli, cooked and chopped

Dissolve broth in water. Add other ingredients and reheat if necessary. Serves 4.

CANTONESE BOUILLON

5 chicken bouillon cubes
4 cups boiling water
1 cup fresh chopped lettuce or watercress
½ cup (small can) water chestnuts, drained and sliced
1 cup bean sprouts, drained
Soy sauce to taste

Dissolve bouillon cubes in water, and simmer watercress or lettuce just until tender. Add remaining ingredients, and simmer 2 minutes more. Serves 5.

RUBY CONSOMMÉ

2 cups tomato juice
2 cups beef consommé
1 tsp soy sauce
1 tsp minced chives
1 tsp lemon juice
⅛ tsp pepper
Sea salt to taste
1 egg white

Bring to boil the tomato juice and beef consommé. Add soy sauce and chives and simmer for 5 minutes. Add lemon juice, pepper and salt. Remove from heat and add gradually to beaten white of an egg. Stir leaving a little foam on the top of the soup, and then pour into bouillon cups. Serves 4.

CRAB MADRILÈNE

1 13-oz can consommé Madrilène
3 oz canned crabmeat, drained and flaked
Sea salt
Pepper
2 tbsp dry sherry
3 slices of lemon
Fresh parsley, chopped

Heat consommé and crab, and season to taste. Remove from heat and add sherry. Serve each cup with a slice of lemon and sprinkling of parsley. Serves 3.

EGG-DROP SOUP

2 eggs
2 tbsp chopped parsley
1 tsp sea salt
½ tsp white pepper
⅛ tsp nutmeg
2 cups chicken bouillon

Beat eggs, parsley, salt, pepper, and nutmeg. Bring bouillon to a full rolling boil. Drop in egg mixture. Serves 2.

BEAN-SPROUT SOUP

6 cups stock or consommé
2 cups chopped bean sprouts
3 eggs, beaten
3 tbsp minced parsley

Heat stock. Add bean sprouts. Simmer about 3 minutes. Remove from heat. Stir in beaten eggs. Sprinkle with parsley. Serves 6.

VEGETABLE-ONION BOUILLON

2 vegetable bouillon cubes
2 cups boiling water
2 medium-sized onions

Dissolve vegetable-broth cubes in boiling water. Slice in onions and cook until tender. Serves 2.

TOMATO-MUSHROOM SOUP

2 8-oz cans mushrooms, drained
2 cups tomato juice
2 cups bouillon
1 tsp garlic salt

Combine all ingredients in saucepan. Cook over low heat, stirring frequently, for 10 minutes or until heated throughout. Serves 4.

"CREAM" OF MUSHROOM SOUP

1 cup well-chopped mushrooms
1 cup condensed consommé
½ cup skim-milk powder
Salt and pepper

Blend skim-milk powder with 2 cups lukewarm water. Cook mushrooms and consommé, covered, until mushrooms are tender. Add to creamy mixture. Season with salt and pepper. Makes 4 servings. Calories in 1 serving: 85.

"CREAM" OF ONION SOUP

¾ cup skim milk
1 tbsp onion flakes
1 chicken bouillon cube *or* 1 packet instant chicken-broth mix

Combine all ingredients in saucepan; cook over low heat, stirring frequently until bouillon cube is dissolved and ingredients are well blended. Serves 1.

GARDEN VEGETABLE BROTH

2 cans (10-12 oz each) condensed beef or chicken broth
2 cups finely chopped fresh vegetables (see Note below)
1 pimiento, finely chopped

Dilute broth with water as directed on label. Heat and add vegetables. Simmer a few minutes and add pimiento. Makes 1½ quarts.

Note: Use any combination of vegetables, such as celery, green pepper, carrots, spinach, watercress, parsley, green onions, and water chestnuts.

Cool Soups for Hot Days

ICED CLAM-TOMATO SOUP

1 cucumber, peeled, seeded, and finely chopped
⅓ cup minced green onion
1 clove garlic, minced
2 cups clam-tomato juice
1 can (15 oz) sliced baby tomatoes
2 tbsp cider vinegar
1 tbsp instant chicken bouillon

Combine all ingredients and chill well before serving. Makes 5 cups.

CURRIED SOUP INDIENNE

3 cups boiling water
4 chicken bouillon cubes
2 tbsp lemon juice
1 egg, well beaten
1 tsp curry powder
Pepper
½ cup leftover turkey or chicken, finely chopped (all
    white meat)
¼ cup seedless green grapes (optional)

Dissolve bouillon cubes in boiling water. Combine lemon juice and egg. Beat in a little hot soup, then a little more. Beat all together. Add curry powder, pepper, and turkey or chicken. Let cool. Add grapes and chill. Serves 4.

QUICK-JELLIED BORSCH

Soften 1 envelope unflavored gelatin in ½ cup water in small saucepan. Heat, stirring constantly, until gelatin dissolves. Stir in 1 can condensed beef broth, 1 can (about 8 oz) diced beets and juice, and 1 tsp prepared horseradish. Pour into a medium-size bowl; chill until softly set. Spoon into chilled cups; top with ¼ cup yogurt and a sprinkling of snipped chives. Serves 4.

JELLIED CHICKEN-VEGETABLE SOUP

1 envelope unflavored gelatin
1 can condensed chicken broth
½ tsp dry mustard
1 tsp Worcestershire
½ cup finely grated carrot
¾ cup minced celery
½ cup minced radishes
Minced chives or green onions

Soften gelatin in ¼ cup cold water. Dissolve over low heat and add to chicken broth with 1 can cold water. Add mustard and Worcestershire, mixed together. Chill to consistency of unbeaten egg white. Then fold in remaining ingredients, except chives. Spoon into 6 individual 5-oz serving dishes and chill. Sprinkle top with chives. Serves 6.

Salads and Vegetables

Keep your salads and vegetables simple while you're reducing.

For a hot vegetable, take your choice of those suggested for salads or any of the eat-all-you-want vegetables, steam lightly and season with herbs suggested on page 56. Or better still, let two large mixed-green and combination salads a day supply your vegetable needs at a low-carbohydrate cost.

Five of my favorite combinations follow the two groups of salad vegetables listed below. Toss with safflower oil and vinegar or lemon juice. Or see the large variety of salad dressings without oil. (Recipes start on page 145.)

I. Take-Your-Choice Greens for Salads

No chance for monotony with such a wide choice. Most of these greens are available in large markets, others in foreign markets, and a few grow wild in regional areas.

Broccoli leaves	Mustard greens
Brussels sprouts leaves	Mustard spinach
Cabbage	Nasturtium leaves and buds
Carrot tops, young	Parsley
Cauliflower leaves	Pepper grass
Celery leaves	Radish tops
Celtuce	Rhubarb leaves
Chicory	Rutabaga tops
Chinese celery	Salsify, young
Collards	Sorrel
Dandelion leaves	Spinach
Endive and escarole	Swiss chard leaves
Fennel	Tampala
Kale	Turnip tops
Kohlrabi leaves	Watercress
Lettuce, all types	Yarrow, young

II. More Take-Your-Choice Salad Vegetables

Artichoke hearts
Asparagus tips, raw, young
Avocado (high in calories, but low in carbohydrate)
Beets, raw, grated, or cut into narrow strips
Broccoli, raw

Brussels sprouts, raw, young, sliced
Carrots, raw, cut in narrow strips or grated
Cauliflower, raw, shredded
Celeriac, raw, diced
Celery, chopped
Cucumber, sliced or diced
Eggplant, raw, diced
Kohlrabi, raw, grated
Onions, all types, sliced, chopped or grated
Peas, tender, young, raw
Peppers, sweet, red and green
Radishes, sliced
Rutabaga, raw, grated or cut into strips
Sprouts, all types
Summer squash, all types, raw, thinly sliced
Tomatoes, all types
Turnips, use same as rutabaga
Water chestnuts, sliced

RABBIT-PATCH SALAD

So crisp and refreshing you won't leave any for the rabbits.

2 cups fresh spinach leaves, broken in bite-sized pieces
2 small cucumbers, sliced
1 cup cherry tomatoes
6 radishes, sliced
4 scallions, sliced
2 carrots, shredded
½ cup celery, sliced
½ head lettuce, broken
2 tbsp fresh parsley, chopped

Toss with oil and vinegar, or your choice of dressings starting on page 145. Serves 6.

ST. PATRICK'S MIXED-GREEN SALAD

Out of County Mayo by way of Brussels, Belgium.

2 heads Belgian endive, sliced
1 cup cabbage, shredded
1 cup fresh spinach leaves, broken into bites
½ head lettuce, broken
½ cup celery, sliced
½ medium onion, in rings
¼ cup green pepper, chopped

Serves 4. (Dressing same as above.)

MIXED GREENS MILANO

As green and colorful as an Italian spring.

½ medium head of escarole
½ medium head of chicory
¼ pound dandelion greens
¼ cup thinly sliced cucumber
¼ cup chopped celery
¼ cup thinly sliced radishes
½ cup wine vinegar
Pinch oregano
Salt and pepper to taste
Safflower or olive oil, if desired

Remove outer leaves from all greens. Tear into 2-inch pieces. Wash and drain on towel. Rub the salad bowl with a cut clove of garlic. Add the remaining ingredients and toss well before serving. Serves 6.

CALICO COLESLAW *

(The recipes starred with an asterisk are those mentioned in my reducing menus in Chapter 4.)

5 cups shredded cabbage
1 tbsp honey
1 tsp sea salt
½ tsp dry mustard
¼ tsp black pepper
¼ cup minced green pepper
¼ cup shredded raw carrots
¼ cup coarsely diced pimientos
½ tsp grated onion
2 tbsp salad oil
⅓ cup cider vinegar

Just before serving: Toss cabbage with honey, salt, mustard, pepper, green pepper, carrots, pimientos and grated onion. In small bowl, combine salad oil and vinegar. Pour over cabbage mixture. Toss well. Serves 6.

FRENCH TOSSED SALAD

(with Roquefort dressing)

1 head of lettuce
A few leaves of romaine lettuce
Additional greens of your choice

2 tomatoes cut into small chunks
½ Bermuda onion, sliced and separated into rings
2 cucumbers sliced thin
1 clove garlic

Rub a wooden salad bowl with a cut clove of garlic. Tear the greens into bite-size pieces. Toss all ingredients in the salad bowl with the following dressing. Serves 6.

Slim-Line Salad Dressings

FRENCH ROQUEFORT DRESSING

4 tbsp vinegar
2 tbsp water
1 clove garlic pressed through a garlic press
½ tsp salt
½ tsp paprika
1 tsp honey
1 tbsp crumbled Roquefort cheese (only a purist would know if you substituted Blue cheese)
1 tbsp chopped chives or scallion greens

Shake up all ingredients in a jar and refrigerate until chilled. Toss with salad just before serving.

"CREAMY" FRENCH DRESSING

⅔ cup creamed cottage cheese
½ cup tomato juice
1 6-oz envelope French salad-dressing mix (or your favorite mixed-herb seasonings)

Mix all ingredients and blend until smooth in blender.

TOMATO FRENCH DRESSING *

1 10¾-oz can condensed tomato soup
¼ tsp garlic powder
¼ tsp onion salt
⅛ tsp black pepper
1 tbsp India relish
2 to 3 tbsp wine vinegar

In a pint jar, shake together tomato soup, garlic powder, onion salt, pepper, relish and vinegar. Cover. Refrigerate until serving time. Makes 1½ cups.

SLIM-LINE BOILED DRESSING

⅔ cup powdered skim milk
¾ tsp unflavored gelatin
1 tsp sea salt
⅛ tsp dry mustard
Dash of Cayenne pepper
1 cup boiling water
2 egg yolks, slightly beaten
2 tbsp lemon juice

Combine dry milk solids, gelatin, salt, dry mustard, and Cayenne pepper in the top of a double boiler. Gradually stir in the boiling water. Slowly add about half the hot mixture to the beaten yolks. Combine thoroughly and return to top of double boiler. Place over boiling water. Cook, stirring constantly, until thickened and smooth. Remove from heat and stir in lemon juice. Cool. Dressing may be stored in refrigerator for several days. Beat with a rotary beater before using. Makes 1½ cups.

EASY YOGURT DRESSING

In a jar combine 2 tsp lemon juice, 1 tbsp salad oil, ½ cup plain yogurt, ½ tsp paprika, dash Tabasco, ½ tsp salt and a pinch of garlic powder. Shake well. Refrigerate. Makes about ⅔ cup.

HERBED YOGURT DRESSING

8 oz plain yogurt
½ to 1 tbsp prepared horseradish
1 tbsp tarragon or garlic vinegar
1 tbsp dried or fresh snipped chives
1 tbsp fresh snipped dill or 1 tsp dried dill weed
¾ tsp sea salt
¼ tsp paprika

In a medium bowl, stir together all ingredients. Cover. Refrigerate until serving time. Dressing may be kept about 3 days. Makes 1 cup.

OLD-FASHIONED BUTTERMILK DRESSING

⅔ cup buttermilk
½ tsp grated lemon rind
2 tsp vinegar

2 tsp chopped fresh chervil
2 tsp chopped fresh tarragon
Sea salt
Pepper

Blend buttermilk with lemon rind and vinegar. Add chervil and tarragon. Season to taste. Let stand 30 minutes. Makes 8 servings. (If fresh herbs are not available, use the dried variety, soaked overnight in the vinegar.)

SLIM-LINE SOUR-CREAM DRESSING

1 cup mock sour cream (see recipe below)
¼ tsp Tabasco
2 tsp horseradish
¼ tsp onion salt
1 tbsp capers
1 tsp minced onion

Combine all ingredients; blend well. Makes 1 cup.

MOCK SOUR CREAM *

Whirl ½ cup creamed cottage cheese and ½ cup buttermilk in blender until smooth. Add 2 tsp lemon juice and whirl a few seconds longer. Makes 1 cup. *Note:* Add chopped chives, if desired.

High Protein at Low Cost

Veal

If your protein budget has been taking a beating and you're tired of spending most of your food money on steak and other costly cuts of beef, here is a variety of succulent veal recipes to help you slim down deliciously and economically. And if you have an old-fashioned cast-iron or stainless steel skillet, you can brown and sauté without oil.

ITALIAN VEAL SCALLOPINI

1 tsp safflower oil
1 lb veal, cut for scallopini
¼ cup dry white wine
1 clove garlic, finely minced

1 4-oz can sliced mushrooms
1 tsp chili sauce
1 beef bouillon cube
1 cup boiling water
1 small bay leaf
⅛ tsp oregano
Garlic salt and pepper

Heat oil in a heavy skillet over moderate heat. Add veal
and brown quickly on both sides. Add wine, garlic, undrained mushrooms, chili sauce, bouillon cube, water, bay
leaf and oregano. Cover tightly and cook over low heat
about 10 minutes. Season to taste with salt and pepper.
Garnish with lemon slices if desired. Serves 4.

HUNGARIAN VEAL PAPRIKA

1½ lb thin veal cutlets
Onion salt
Pepper
1 tbsp paprika
2 tbsp lemon juice
½ cup catsup
½ cup yogurt or mock sour cream

Brown cutlets in heavy iron or stainless steel skillet, and
cook 5 to 7 minutes. Drain off any fat. Sprinkle with salt,
pepper, and paprika. Combine lemon juice, catsup and
sour cream. Pour over and simmer gently 5 more minutes.
Serves 6.

CURRIED VEAL BOMBAY

1 lb lean veal cut into ¾-inch cubes
1½ tsp cooking oil
1 small onion, chopped
1 tsp curry powder
Dash ginger
¼ tsp cinnamon
⅛ tsp turmeric
⅛ tsp paprika
½ tsp sea salt
1 cup fat-free chicken broth
½ green pepper, seeded and slivered
½ red pepper, seeded and slivered

Make sure veal is trimmed of all fat. Heat oil in a skillet
and sauté veal, a few pieces at a time until golden on all

sides. Push meat to one side, add onion and sauté until pale gold. Add all seasonings and stir for a few minutes over heat. Add chicken broth and simmer about 1 hour or until veal is almost tender. Add green and red peppers and continue simmering until veal is tender. Peppers should be crisp tender. To thicken liquid a little more, cook uncovered for a few minutes. Serves 4.

SCANDINAVIAN POT ROAST

    1 6-lb boned and rolled veal rump roast
    3 tbsp safflower oil
    2 cups yogurt
    1 package onion-soup mix
    2 tsp dill seed
    1 tsp onion or sea salt
    ¼ tsp pepper

In Dutch oven over medium-high heat, in hot oil, brown roast on all sides. In small bowl, combine yogurt, onion-soup mix, dill, salt and pepper; spoon over roast. Cover pan and simmer over low heat 2½ to 3 hours, or until veal is fork-tender. Serves 12-14. (For smaller servings, reduce ingredients proportionately.)

SKILLET VEAL CHOPS WITH PIMIENTOS

    6 loin veal chops
    Salt and pepper
    ½ tsp oregano
    2 medium onions, sliced
    1 can (4 oz) sliced mushrooms, undrained
    1 cup chicken broth
    1 jar (4 oz) pimientos, drained and chopped

Brown chops on both sides in hot skillet. Season with salt and pepper and oregano. Add onions, mushrooms with liquid and broth. Cover and simmer 20 minutes. Add pimientos and simmer 10 more minutes. Serves 6.

Earlier in this chapter I promised you two of Mrs. Mattison's Parisian veal recipes. Here they are, with her suggestions for accompanying vegetables. (No measurements were given, but none are necessary. The recipes are elegant, but simple to prepare.)

LONGE DE VEAU À LA GENDARME

Lard a loin of veal lengthwise with pistachio nuts and thin strips of smoked beef tongue, with the help of a skewer. Brown it in the oven with herbs, moistened with port wine and veal stock. When the meat is done, strain the juices and thicken slightly. Slice across the direction of the larding so that each slice is sprinkled with little dots of red and green. Serve with oven-baked tomatoes, and braised lettuce hearts. Could also be served with purée of celery.

LONGE DE VEAU SOUBISE

Brown loin of veal in a casserole until it is golden—cover and cook until done. When it is done, cut it in slices and spread each slice with a purée of onions. Cover the reshaped loin of veal with more onion purée, sprinkle with grated cheese, and brown in the oven. Serve with celery hearts and carrots sprinkled with parsley. Use the stock from the veal as an accompanying sauce. Could also be served with watercress purée, which is excellent with veal.

STUFFED VEAL BIRDS

Back to America for a finale of versatile veal recipes. Remember the homey-good veal birds of childhood days? They've been brought up to date with a slim-line stuffing of broccoli instead of bread.

    4 slices (¾ lb) veal scallops, ¼-inch thick
    Sea salt and white pepper
    Grated rind of 1 lemon
    4 broccoli spears
    1 can (10-12 oz) condensed chicken broth
    1½ tbsp tomato paste
    Minced parsley

Season veal slices lightly with salt and pepper. Sprinkle with lemon rind. Place a raw broccoli spear on top of each. Roll up and fasten with toothpick. Combine chicken broth with tomato paste in small skillet. Bring to boil and simmer a few minutes. Add veal rolls, cover and simmer 15 to 20 minutes, or until meat is tender. Remove toothpicks. Sprinkle with parsley. Serves 4.

POTTED VEAL WITH VEGETABLES

1 boned shoulder of veal (approx. 4 lbs)
2 tsp seasoned salt
¼ tsp seasoned pepper
½ tsp thyme
2 tbsp safflower oil
1½ cups canned chicken broth
8 large carrots, quartered
1½ lb fresh green beans, cleaned, left whole
Snipped parsley for garnish

Unroll shoulder of veal; trim all extra fat from meat; sprinkle it with seasoned salt, seasoned pepper, and thyme; roll it up again, and then tie with string. In hot oil, in large Dutch oven, brown veal on all sides; add chicken broth and simmer, covered, about 1½ hours. Now add quartered carrots, cook them 10 minutes, then add green beans and continue cooking until both vegetables and veal are tender. Thinly slice veal into serving portions. Sprinkle with parsley. Serves 8.

VEAL RAGOUT WITH WINE

Cooking with wine can turn a homespun dish into party fare. Heat evaporates the alcohol, so your chances of getting either fat or intoxicated go up in steam, leaving only the flavor.

2½ lb very lean veal, cut into 1-inch cubes
2 onions, diced
1 clove garlic, pressed
2 cups dry white wine
1 tsp oregano
1 tsp thyme
2 bay leaves
4 tomatoes, peeled and coarsely chopped
1 tsp onion salt
Pepper
2 4-oz cans sliced mushrooms and liquid

Brown veal in skillet. Remove to kettle. Drain off any fat, and cook onions and garlic until limp. Add these to kettle. Add mushrooms' liquid and remaining ingredients except for drained mushrooms. Cover and simmer 1 hour. Add mushrooms, and continue cooking until they're just heated. Serves 8.

Lamb

LAMB SHANKS MEDITERRANEAN *

This is the only lamb recipe included on my own reducing diet. It's one of my favorites, though for the most part I feel that you get too much fat and too little value in lamb to recommend it on a restricted diet.

4 to 6 lamb shanks
½ clove garlic, cut in small pieces
1 tsp sea salt
½ tsp pepper
1 tsp paprika
2 tbsp safflower oil
1 bay leaf, crushed
4 whole black peppers
1 tbsp grated lemon rind
½ cup lemon juice
1 lemon, cut in wedges

Make small gashes in lamb shanks and insert a piece of garlic in each. Season with the salt, pepper and paprika. In heavy kettle or Dutch oven brown shanks slowly in the oil. Then add 1 cup water and remaining ingredients, except lemon wedges. Bring to boil, cover and simmer 2 to 2¼ hours, or until meat is very tender. Turn meat occasionally and baste with pan drippings. Serve with lemon wedges. Serves 4 to 6.

Chicken

Broiling is a fine, nonfattening way to cook chicken, but it does spatter up the broiler. And fried chicken—which is too fattening, anyway!—spatters the cooks and sometimes the ceiling. Here are some easy, economical ways with chicken that will slim you down without spattering you up.

OVEN-BROILED CHICKEN

1 chicken, quartered
2 tbsp wheat germ
Sea salt and pepper to taste
Paprika

Remove skin from chicken. Place in baking pan, bone side down. Sprinkle each piece with wheat germ. Cover pan tightly with foil. Bake 30 minutes at 350°. Remove foil and broil for ten minutes, or until it starts to brown. Sprinkle with salt, pepper, and paprika. Serves 4.

BAKED CHICKEN, ORIENTAL

2 broiler-fryer chickens, quartered
1 tsp sea salt
½ cup prepared mustard
2 tbsp vinegar
2 tbsp water
2 tbsp safflower oil
1 tsp dried leaf thyme
¼ tsp ginger

Sprinkle chicken on both sides with salt. Place skin side up in foil-lined shallow baking pan. Mix together mustard, vinegar, water, oil, thyme and ginger. Spoon over chicken. Bake in 375°F oven 50 to 60 minutes. Serves 8.

BARBECUED CHICKEN CHINESE STYLE

¼ cup soy sauce
1 tbsp safflower oil
¾ tsp dry mustard
¼ tsp ground ginger
⅛ tsp pepper
1 small clove garlic, minced
1 frying chicken, quartered

Mix all ingredients, except chicken. Put chicken in shallow baking pan and brush on all sides with the mixture. Let stand 30 minutes. Then bake in moderate oven (350°F) 50 minutes, or until tender, turning once or twice and brushing with the sauce. Serves 4.

CHICKEN À LA GRECQUE*

1 3-lb broiler-fryer chicken, skinned, cut up
Paprika
Garlic salt
¼ tsp black pepper
2 tbsp safflower oil
½ cup canned chicken broth
1 clove garlic
1 medium eggplant, pared, cubed
1 medium onion, peeled, chopped

2 tomatoes, peeled, diced
¼ tsp thyme
1 tbsp snipped parsley

Sprinkle chicken pieces with paprika, 1 tsp salt and pepper. In oil in large skillet, sauté chicken until golden. Stir in broth, scraping brown particles from bottom of skillet. Stick toothpick into garlic, then add to skillet with eggplant, onion, tomatoes, thyme, parsley, 1 tsp salt. Simmer, covered, 30 minutes or until chicken is tender. Remove garlic. Serves 6.

BAKED CHICKEN WITH MOCK SOUR CREAM

1 2½- to 3-lb broiler-fryer chicken, cut in half
6 tbsp mock sour cream
2 tbsp lemon juice
½ tsp crushed dried rosemary leaves
¼ tsp sea salt
Dash of pepper
4 tsp wheat germ
Dash of paprika
1 tbsp parsley

Heat oven to 375°F. Wash and dry chicken. Blend sour cream, lemon juice, rosemary, salt and pepper. Spread half the sour-cream mixture over chicken and arrange in a shallow baking dish; bake uncovered about 50 minutes, or until fork-tender. Brush with remaining sour-cream mixture. Sprinkle with wheat germ and paprika; continue to bake 10 minutes longer. Garnish with parsley. Serves 4.

CHICKEN CACCIATORE

1 frying chicken (about 3 lbs) cut up
¼ cup safflower oil
2 onions, sliced
2 cloves garlic, crushed
1 can (1 lb) Italian-style tomatoes
1 can (8 oz) tomato sauce
1 tsp sea salt
¼ tsp pepper
1 tsp crushed dried oregano leaves
2 bay leaves
Italian-style grated cheese

Brown chicken on all sides in the hot oil in large deep skillet. Remove chicken and keep warm. Cook onion and

garlic in oil remaining in skillet until lightly browned. Add
remaining ingredients, except cheese, and simmer 5 minutes. Put chicken back in skillet and cook, covered, 45
minutes or until tender. Arrange chicken on hot platter,
skim excess fat from sauce and remove bay leaves; pour
over chicken. Serve with cheese. Serves 4.

ORANGE-HERB CHICKEN

1 2¾-lb broiler-fryer chicken cut in pieces
Pepper
Paprika
3 tbsp fresh parsley, chopped
½ tsp rosemary
¼ cup orange juice

Heat oven to 325°F. Rub or sprinkle chicken with next 4
ingredients. Place skin down on broiler pan, or other pan
that allows for draining. Pour orange juice slowly and
evenly over. Bake 45 minutes. Turn skin side up and bake
15 minutes more. Serves 4.

OVEN-FRIED CHICKEN

1 chicken (about 2½ lbs) quartered
¼ cup evaporated skim milk
Sea salt and pepper
½ cup wheat germ
¾ tsp crushed rosemary leaves

Dip chicken pieces in the milk and sprinkle both sides with
salt and pepper. Dip in wheat germ mixed with rosemary,
coating both sides. Arrange chicken pieces on rack in
shallow baking pan. Add water to pan to depth of ¼ inch.
Bake in moderate oven (350°F) 1 hour, or until tender.
Serves 4.

CHICKEN PAPRIKA

1 fryer chicken, about 3½ lbs, cut up
1 tsp onion salt
¼ tsp white pepper
Pinch of cayenne
3 tbsp olive or safflower oil
1 medium onion, thinly sliced

> 1 clove garlic, minced
> 1 cup mock sour cream or yogurt
> 3 to 4 tsp paprika

Season chicken with the salt, pepper and Cayenne. Heat oil in heavy skillet with cover and brown chicken well. Remove. Add onion and garlic and sauté until onion is golden. Add chicken and sour cream and sprinkle paprika over top. Cover and simmer gently 30 to 35 minutes, or until chicken is done. Pour sauce over chicken when serving. Serves 4.

CHICKEN AND LOBSTER CANTONESE

(Or what to do with leftover chicken or turkey)

> 1½ cups (7 oz) leftover turkey or chicken
> 1 6½-oz can lobster, drained
> 1 tbsp safflower oil
> 1 clove garlic, minced (optional)
> 1 green pepper, cut in strips
> 1 small onion, sliced
> 1 cup celery, diced
> ½ cup boiling water
> 1 chicken bouillon cube
> ½ cup (small can) water chestnuts, drained and sliced
> 2 cups bean sprouts, drained
> 2 tbsp soy sauce
> ¼ tsp ginger
> Pepper

Heat oil in skillet, tilting pan to coat bottom. Sauté garlic, green pepper, onion and celery. Dissolve bouillon cube in water, and add. Cover, and simmer 8 to 10 minutes. Add chicken, lobster, and all remaining ingredients and simmer an additional 5 minutes. If necessary add a little more water. Serves 6.

HERBED BAKED CHICKEN
WITH MUSHROOMS

> 2 broiler-fryer chickens, quartered
> 2 tsp celery salt
> 1 tsp celery seed
> ½ tsp dried leaf marjoram
> 1 can (6 or 8 oz) mushrooms

Sprinkle chicken quarters with salt. Place skin side up in shallow baking pan. Sprinkle with celery seed and marjoram. Add liquid from mushrooms. Bake in 375°F oven 30 minutes; spoon liquid in pan over chicken occasionally. Add mushrooms. Bake 20 to 30 minutes longer, until chicken is tender. Serve with Hungarian Sauerkraut (recipe follows).

HUNGARIAN SAUERKRAUT *

1 lb. sauerkraut, drained
1 tbsp caraway seeds
½ cup tomato juice

Mix sauerkraut with caraway seeds and tomato juice. Simmer slowly in tightly covered pan until sauerkraut is tender and tomato juice is well absorbed. Serves 4.

Fish and Seafood

If you're fond of fish, dieting should be easy for you. High in protein and minerals from the sea and kind to your taste buds and budget, it can speed up your slimming-down program. Have it often.

BAKED FISH *

(Basic Recipe)
With cottage cheese and chive sauce

1 lb fish (haddock, flounder, or sole) fillets
Sea salt and pepper to taste
½ cup creamed cottage cheese
½ tbsp skimmed milk
2 tbsp prepared horseradish
1 tbsp lemon juice
2 tsp snipped chives

Preheat oven to 450°F. Salt and pepper each side of fish fillets, then place in lightly oiled shallow baking dish. Tightly cover dish and bake for 15 to 20 minutes, or until fish flakes. Meanwhile place cottage cheese, milk, horse-radish, and lemon juice in an electric-blender container; blend at low speed until a smooth sauce; stir in chives. (Or cottage cheese may be pressed through a fine sieve and mixed with other ingredients.) Heat sauce and serve over fish. Serves 3-4.

HERBED BAKED FISH

With wheat germ

1½ lb fish fillets
½ tsp sea salt
⅛ tsp pepper
¼ tsp ground thyme
½ tsp tarragon leaves
2 tbsp instant minced onion
1 small clove garlic, minced
1 cup tomato juice
½ cup wheat germ

Sprinkle fish with salt, pepper, and thyme. Fold each fillet loosely into thirds; place in baking dish. Add tarragon, onion, and garlic to tomato juice. Slowly pour over fish. Sprinkle wheat germ over fish. Bake at 400°F (hot oven) for 8 minutes, or until fish flakes easily with fork. Serves 4-6.

FILLET OF SOLE ITALIAN

¼ cup chopped onion
2 cups sliced fresh mushrooms
1 tbsp safflower oil
2 lb sole fillets
2 tbsp lemon juice
1 tbsp chopped parsley
1 tsp oregano
¼ tsp pepper

In a large skillet sauté onions and mushrooms in oil until tender. Layer sole in pan and sprinkle remaining ingredients over fish. Cover and simmer for 20 minutes. Serves 6-8.

POACHED HALIBUT

With Cucumber-Dill Sauce

1½ lb fish fillets, cut into 4 serving pieces
1 tbsp safflower oil
3 tbsp minced onion
¼ cup buttermilk
½ tsp onion salt
Pepper
Water

Heat oil in skillet. Sauté onion until limp. Add remaining

ingredients, using enough water to bring the pan level up to ½ inch. Cover with foil, with a small steam hole cut in the center. Simmer 5 to 10 minutes, until fish is fork-tender. Serve with:

CUCUMBER-DILL SAUCE

1 large cucumber, grated
1 cup yogurt (or mock sour cream)
1 tbsp lemon juice
½ tsp prepared mustard
½ tsp dill salt

Combine all ingredients mixing well, and refrigerate until ready to use.

BROILED SALMON, PARISIAN

1 lb salmon steaks
½ tsp sea salt
Dash pepper
½ tsp rosemary leaves
1 tbsp wine vinegar
2 tbsp safflower oil

Sprinkle both sides of steaks with salt and pepper. Add rosemary and vinegar to the salad oil; shake well, and let stand at room temperature for an hour or longer; strain. Dip fish in oil mixture, and place on a preheated oiled broiler pan about 2 inches from the heat. Broil 5 to 8 minutes or until slightly brown. Baste with oil, and turn carefully. Brush other side with oil, and cook 5 to 8 minutes more or until fish flakes easily when tested with a fork. Serve immediately. Serves 4.

LA COSTA CASSOLETTE OF SCALLOPS

From another fabulous reducing spa, La Costa, between Los Angeles and San Diego, comes a celebrity-slimming recipe enjoyed by such stars as Lucille Ball, Janet Leigh, Dinah Shore, and many others.

12 sea scallops
¼ cup fresh lemon juice
1 tbsp white wine
4 sliced fresh mushrooms

1 tbsp chopped shallots
1 medium-size tomato (scald, peel and dice)
¼ cup clam juice
½ cup chopped parsley

Wash scallops. Drain carefully to remove any sand. Pre-heat broiler so it is very hot. Place the scallops in a small, heat-proof casserole and squeeze lemon juice over them. Broil 2 minutes, shaking to turn juices. Turn scallops, but do not pierce them with a fork. When all are turned, add wine to casserole, then mushrooms, shallots, tomato and clam juice. Cover. Simmer on top of stove 7-10 minutes. Garnish with finely chopped parsley and serve. Serves 2.

LOUISIANA SHRIMP

1 green pepper, chopped
¾ cup celery, diced
½ cup onion, diced
1½ cups canned tomatoes
½ cup water
¼ cup lemon juice
1 tsp onion or sea salt
½ tsp oregano
Pepper
1½ lb cooked shrimp

Combine first 9 ingredients, and simmer until vegetables are tender, about 7 to 10 minutes. Add shrimp, and cook 3 minutes more. Serves 6.

NIPPY SHRIMP, NIPPONESE

1 tbsp safflower oil
1 lb shelled and deveined medium shrimp
2 tbsp soy sauce
2 tbsp vinegar
2 tbsp catsup
½ tsp ginger
½ tsp garlic salt
2 scallions, chopped

In medium skillet over low heat, in oil, sauté shrimp 4 minutes. Add remaining ingredients; simmer 5 minutes. Serves 4.

LOBSTER CANTONESE *

With bean sprouts and celery

3 lobsters (1 lb each) split lengthwise
2 tbsp soya sauce
1 tsp sherry
1 small onion, finely chopped
2 tbsp water

Steam lobsters over boiling water. On each lobster half pour soya sauce, sherry, onion, and water mixed. Continue steaming for 10 minutes. Serves 6.

BEANSPROUTS WITH CELERY*

Sauté 3 stalks chopped celery, 1 small chopped onion, 6 sliced mushrooms in safflower oil. Add 1 lb beansprouts, 1 tbsp each of soya sauce and water, and 1 tsp salt. Stir 5 minutes and simmer.

Fish-and-Egg Combinations

Good for breakfast, luncheons, or a light dinner. The first two are breakfast favorites of mine.

SALMON-EGG PATTY WITH WHEAT GERM *

1 7-oz can red salmon
2 eggs, beaten
1 cup wheat germ
1 tbsp grated onion
Pinch of basil
1 tsp safflower oil

Remove skin and bone from salmon. Add wheat germ, beaten eggs, onion and basil. Blend well. Form into patties and sauté in lightly oiled skillet over medium heat until golden-brown. Serves 3 or 4.

BAKED EGGS WITH ANCHOVIES *

1 can anchovies
1 cup Mock Sour Cream (page 147)
¼ lb mushrooms, sliced
2 tsp safflower oil

2 tbsp chopped parsley
Freshly ground pepper
4 eggs
¼ cup grated Parmesan cheese

Chop anchovies, add to mock sour cream and mix well. Turn into lightly oiled 4-cup baking dish and bake in preheated 400° oven until mixture begins to bubble.

Sauté mushrooms in oil until soft. Add mushrooms and parsley to sour-cream mixture. Continue baking until mixture is reduced by about a third. Season to taste with pepper. Turn off oven heat. Remove baking dish from oven, closing oven door to retain heat. Break each egg into a saucer and slide carefully into the sauce. Sprinkle with grated cheese, return to lowest part of the oven and cook gently until eggs are set. Serves 4.

SHRIMP FOO YONG

6 eggs
6 tbsp chopped bamboo shoots
6 tbsp chopped water chestnuts
6 tbsp shredded Chinese pea pods (snow peas)
1 cup bean sprouts
¾ cup finely chopped shrimp

Mix all the vegetables and shrimp and fold in with the beaten eggs. Sauté in oil about 5 minutes. Serves 4.

Beef Budget-Savers

If you can cook at all, you know how to broil steak and, like most of us, probably have it as often as your budget permits. When it doesn't, here are a few low-cost beef recipes I have enjoyed both at home and in other countries.

DILLED MEAT BALLS, FINLANDIA

1 lb ground beef
½ cup wheat germ
½ cup minced onion
¼ cup minced green pepper
1½ tsp dill or onion weed
¾ tsp salt
2 tbsp safflower oil
1 8-oz can tomato sauce

¼ cup chopped dill pickles
1 tbsp Worcestershire
½ cup water

In medium bowl, mix ground beef, wheat germ, onion, green pepper, dill and salt; shape into 2-inch balls. Using large skillet, brown balls in hot oil, over medium-high heat. Add tomato sauce, pickles, and Worcestershire and water. Simmer covered 35 minutes. Serves 4.

SKILLET-BURGER LOAF*

1 lb ground round steak
1 egg
¾ tsp onion or sea salt
2 tbsp instant minced onions
3 Cheddar cheese slices
¼ tsp black pepper
Snipped parsley (for garnish)

Combine ground meat, egg, salt, and instant minced onion. Oil an 8-inch skillet; lightly pat one half of meat over bottom of it; arrange cheese slices on top. Cover with rest of meat, patting smooth. Sprinkle with pepper; cut into 4 pie-shaped wedges. Cook, on top of range, over fairly high heat, until browned on bottom. Turn, brown other side, and cook until done as desired. Garnish with parsley. Serves 4.

RUSSIAN HIGH-PROTEIN MEAT LOAF

2 cups creamed cottage chese
3 cups cooked millet meal
½ cup yogurt
1½ lb lean ground beef
½ cup wheat germ
½ cup finely chopped onion
½ cup finely chopped celery
½ cup catsup
4 tsp vegetable salt
⅛ tsp pepper
2 eggs, beaten

Beat cottage cheese until almost smooth. Add remaining ingredients and mix together thoroughly. Oil a loaf pan with safflower oil and press mixture into it. Bake 1 hour 15 minutes in moderately hot oven (350°). Serves 8.

(Millet meal—ground millet seed—is available in health food stores.)

ORIENTAL HAMBURGERS

1 lb round steak or chuck, ground
1 onion, minced
½ cup finely chopped sprouts
1 clove garlic, minced
½ cup soy sauce
¼ tsp ground ginger

Mix beef, onion, and sprouts. Shape into 4 patties. Place in shallow dish. Mix remaining ingredients. Pour over patties. Let stand 30 minutes, turning patties once. Drain, and broil or sauté to desired doneness. Serves 4.

TERIYAKI STEAK, HAWAIIAN

2 lb lean round steak, cut at least ¾-inch thick
2 or 3 small pieces gingerroot, crushed with a hammer
1 clove garlic, pressed
½ cup soy sauce
1½ tbsp honey

Combine marinade ingredients, and pour over steak. Marinate in refrigerator 6 to 8 hours, turning steak occasionally. Remove from marinade (which is a fine tenderizer for all cuts of meat), drain, and broil. Serves 6.

CHUCK STEAK ITALIAN

2 lb chuck steak
Papaya meat tenderizer
1 can (1 lb) tomatoes
½ tsp oregano
1 tbsp minced onion
1 clove garlic, minced
1 tsp minced parsley
Garlic salt and pepper
2 tbsp safflower oil or olive oil
1 tbsp grated Parmesan cheese

Cut meat into serving pieces. Sprinkle with papaya tenderizer. Let stand ½ hour for each ½-inch thickness of meat. (If time is short, use instant tenderizer.) Arrange meat in original shape in a baking dish, not too large, into which the meat fits compactly. With a fork, break canned tomatoes into pieces. Drain off half the juice and reserve it. Combine tomatoes, oregano, onion, garlic, parsley, salt and pepper. Pour over meat. Pour oil evenly over all. Bake uncovered about 1½ hours in 350° oven. Add some of the reserved tomato juice if bottom of pan gets dry or starts to char. For last 15 minutes of cooking sprinkle with Parmesan cheese. Serves 4-6.

FRENCH BEEF STEW

2½ lb lean round steak, cubed
8 carrots, chunked
6 stalks celery, sliced
2 large onions, diced
1 green pepper, in chunks
2 tsp sea salt
1 tsp rosemary
1 tsp sweet basil
1 tsp thyme
1 cup red wine
3 cups water
Pepper
Fresh parsley, chopped

Brown meat in iron skillet, using small amount of safflower oil. Remove to stewing kettle. Drain off oil, and sauté onions and green pepper in skillet. Add to kettle. Add remaining ingredients, except parsley, and bring to a boil. Cover and simmer slowly 1½ to 2 hours. Garnish with parsley. Serves 8.

ENGLISH STEAK-AND-KIDNEY STEW

1 lb lamb kidneys, cleaned and sliced
1 lb lean round steak, cut in strips
1½ cups dry red wine
1 tsp sea salt
2 bay leaves
2 onions, chopped
4 carrots, sliced
2 4-oz cans sliced mushrooms
Pepper
3 tbsp fresh parsley, chopped
11½ cups water

Marinate meat in wine, with salt and bay leaf added, for 1 hour. Remove from marinade, and brown meat in skillet. Remove meat and drain off fat. Cook onion, until just limp. Combine wine marinade, meat, and onions in kettle.

Add remaining ingredients, except for mushrooms and parsley. Bring to a boil, then simmer, covered, 1½ hours. Add mushrooms and liquid and cook 5 minutes more. Season with pepper and garnish with parsley. Serves 6.

Liver Is Important for Slimmers

Nutrition-paced and low in cost, low in calories, low in fat—liver belongs on your table often, whether you're dieting or not. This excellent organ meat had a prominent place in my own reducing diet. If you have an aversion for this highly nutritious food, do try to learn to like it. The benefits are tremendous.

Calves' liver, liver from young spring lamb, and chicken livers need very little cooking. They are tender and delicious when just heated through and lightly browned, either under the broiler, panbroiled, or sautéed in a skillet lightly oiled with just enough safflower oil to prevent sticking.

Liver from older animals (beef, mutton, or older lamb) may be cooked the same way if the slices are first tenderized by marinating them for 10 minutes, and then dried and cooked as desired. Cooking liver in a covered pan or by one of the moist-heat methods, such as braising, also will tenderize the less-tender slices.

Do not soak liver. Wash it as little as possible, preferably with a damp cloth.

Trim liver as needed, with curved scissors or a sharp knife, and remove membrane.

To retain the flavor, the tenderness and extraordinary vitamin content of liver, cook it at a low temperature—and do not overcook.

BROILED LIVER

Because it's low in fat, liver (and other organ meats) can be broiled without spattering grease on your broiler.

For broiling, liver should be at least ⅓-inch thick. Place liver on broiling rack, about 3 inches from moderate heat. Leave door of broiling oven open. Broil liver for a total of 2 minutes: 1 minute for each side. Season to taste with flavored salt, pepper, and paprika. If desired, top with slices of broiled onion. Or dot with butter, a sprinkle of lemon juice, and chopped parsley.

QUICK CHICKEN LIVERS

1 tbsp safflower oil
2 large onions, cut in thin slices
2 large stalks green celery, thinly sliced
1 lb fresh chicken livers (or frozen livers, thawed)
Sea salt
Pepper
Garlic powder (optional)

About 15 minutes before serving: Using a large skillet, sauté onion and celery slices in oil until onion is just wilted. Push onions to one side; turn up heat to a high setting. Add chicken livers; top with onions; then cook, turning livers once or twice, until done as you like them— 3 to 5 minutes. Season to taste with sea salt, pepper, and garlic powder. Serves 3.

CHICKEN-LIVER KEBOBS

1 lb chicken livers
2 medium onions
1 green pepper
8 medium fresh mushrooms
1 tbsp safflower oil

If chicken livers are large, cut them in half. Cut each onion into 4 wedges; the green pepper, into 8 chunks. Alternate livers and vegetables on skewers. Brush with oil. Broil, turning once or twice, until livers are golden-brown. Serves 4.

BRAISED BEEF LIVER AND MUSHROOMS

1 lb beef liver, cut into 4 equal slices
¼ cup sliced onions
1 4-oz can sliced mushrooms, undrained
¼ cup dry sherry
2 tbsp chopped parsley
1 tbsp lemon juice
½ tsp sea salt
⅛ tsp pepper

Heat oil in a skillet over moderately low heat (about 225°F). Brown liver on both sides and add remaining ingredients. Cover and cook 10 minutes, or until liver is done. Serves 4.

Desserts, or Aren't You Fat Enough, Anyway?

Just about the best slimming advice I can give you is to stick to fresh fruit, melon, berries, or cheese for dessert.

No, there isn't a shortage of dessert recipes for dieters. The trouble is, I can't in good conscience recommend those loaded with artificial sweeteners, and most of them are.

Here are a few of the exceptions that you may have occasionally. Just don't expect to lose weight if you eat them at every meal. And do keep the portions moderate or you'll stop losing and start gaining.

The first two recipes are slightly modified versions of desserts served at the Golden Door and La Costa reducing spas.

GOLDEN DOOR FRESH STRAWBERRY RING

    1 envelope unflavored gelatin
    ½ cup cold water
    2 cups (1 pint) fresh strawberries
    1 tsp lemon juice
    2 egg whites
    ¼ cup honey

Soften gelatin in water in a small saucepan. Heat slowly, stirring constantly, until gelatin dissolves; remove from heat; cool. Wash strawberries; hull. Crush coarsely in a medium-size bowl; stir in gelatin mixture and lemon juice. Chill until as thick as unbeaten egg white.

Beat egg whites until foamy-white and double in volume in a small bowl; beat in honey *1 tbsp at a time*, beating all the time until meringue stands in firm peaks. Fold into thickened strawberry mixture until no streaks of white remain. Spoon into a 4-cup tube mold. Chill several hours, or until firm. Unmold. Garnish with whole strawberries. Serves 6. (Unsweetened frozen strawberries may be used if fresh are not available.)

ORANGE ALASKA LA COSTA

Select small, sweet oranges. Slice off one-third from the stem end and set it aside. Remove pulp, catching juice in a bowl. Place juice and pulp in blender. Whir 1 minute. Refrigerate shells. Pour juice into ice-cube trays and when almost solid, beat with rotary or electric mixer till it reaches sherbet consistency. Refreeze and beat again. Fill orange cups. Beat 1 egg white till frothy, add ¼ tsp vanilla extract, 2 tsp honey, and beat till stiff. Top orange cup with meringuelike garnish. Set under broiler 6 inches from heat until golden brown—approximately 3-5 minutes. (One egg white will frost 2 orange shells.) Serve at once.

STRAWBERRY YOGURT FREEZE

    1 cup plain yogurt
    2 cups fresh strawberries, halved
    ⅓ cup honey
    1 tbsp lemon juice

Whirl all ingredients in blender until smooth. Pour into ice-cube tray and freeze until firm around edges. Turn into chilled bowl and beat until smooth. Put back in tray and freeze until firm. Let stand at room temperature to soften slightly before serving. Serves 3.

Variation:

Substitute fresh peaches or other fresh fruit for strawberries. (Unsweetened frozen strawberries may be used if fresh are not available.)

PINEAPPLE-MINT FRAPPÉ

    1 can (1 lb, 4 oz) pineapple chunks in pure juice
    2 tbsp coarsely chopped mint leaves

Set aside 4 pineapple chunks for garnish. Turn remaining pineapple and the liquid into a 9-inch square pan. Place in freezer until almost completely frozen—will take about 1½ hours. Turn into electric blender, along with chopped mint; cover; blend at low speed just until smooth, but not melted. Spoon into 4 sherbert glasses. Top each frappé with a reserved pineapple chunk and a sprig of mint if desired. Serves 4.

QUICK PINEAPPLE SHERBET

Freeze 1 can (20 oz) pineapple chunks packed in unsweetened juice, until solidly frozen. Put under running hot water 1 minute before opening. Then put frozen chunks in blender and whirl. Stop blender occasionally and with wooden or rubber spatula work fruit into sherbet consistency. Serves 4.

Variation:

Mint-pineapple sherbet. Blend about 20 fresh mint leaves with the pineapple. Top each serving with a sprig of mint.

PINEAPPLE YOGURT SHERBET

1 cup yogurt
1 tbsp lemon juice
½ cup pineapple juice (unsweetened)
¼ cup crushed pineapple
1 tbsp honey
2 egg whites

Mix yogurt, lemon juice, pineapple juice, pineapple, and honey thoroughly. Put in freezer tray and freeze until firm. Then take it out, put it in a bowl and stir until mixture is smooth and free of lumps. Beat egg whites until stiff. Fold them into the smooth creamy mixture. Return to freezer tray and freeze. Serves 3-4.

Variations:

Orange sherbet: Substitute fresh or canned orange juice for pineapple juice, and orange-juice concentrate for crushed pineapple.

Apricot sherbet: Substitute apricot nectar for pineapple juice, and puréed canned or cooked apricots for crushed pineapple.

SLIM-LINE VANILLA ICE CREAM

½ cup skim milk powder
1½ cups water
3 tsp honey
1½ tsp vanilla
1 envelope unflavored gelatin
1 tbsp cold water

Thoroughly mix milk powder with water to make extra strength reconstituted milk. Pour into saucepan with honey and vanilla. Heat over low flame until just warm, not hot. Remove from heat. Dissolve gelatin in cold water; add to warm milk. Stir until well-mixed. Pour into freezer tray. Let stand at room temperature about 10 minutes.

Place in refrigerator freezer section. Turn dial to highest speed. Freeze until firm. Remove from tray to chilled bowl. Beat until smooth. Return to freezer tray. Freeze until ready to serve. About 6 portions.
Variations:

For coffee flavor, add 2 tbsp instant powdered coffee to warm-milk mixture before heating. For chocolate-like flavor, add ¼ cup carob powder.

CHIFFON DESSERT

  1 envelope unflavored gelatin
  2 tbsp honey
  ⅛ tsp sea salt
  3 egg yolks
  1¼ cups fresh whole or skim milk
  1 tsp vanilla extract
  ¼ tsp nutmeg
  3 egg whites

Mix gelatin, honey and salt in top of double boiler. Beat together egg yolks and fresh milk. Add to gelatin mixture. Cook over boiling water, stirring constantly until gelatin is dissolved, about 5 minutes. Remove from heat; add vanilla and nutmeg. Chill until mixture thickens slightly. Beat egg whites until stiff and fold in gelatin mixture. Turn into molds and chill until firm. Serves 6.
Variations:

"Chocolate" chiffon: Add ⅓ cup carob powder; double the honey, eliminate nutmeg. (Carob powder, which looks like and tastes like chocolate, is low in starch, rich in calcium and has only 2 percent fat. Chocolate has 52 percent fat.)

Orange chiffon: Reduce milk to ¾ cup; add ¾ cup orange juice and grated rind of 1 orange. Instead of vanilla use lemon extract.

Pineapple chiffon: Add ½ cup crushed pineapple. Omit vanilla and nutmeg.

Crustless Pies

BLUEBERRY CHEESE PIE

  1½ cup small-curd cottage cheese
  1 cup blueberries, drained if canned or frozen

⅓ cup honey
2 eggs
1 lemon, grated rind and juice
2 tbsp cream
½ tsp cinnamon
2 tbsp safflower oil

Press cheese through sieve or ricer. Beat eggs, add honey and other ingredients. Pour into pastry-lined pie pan or well-oiled 8-inch glass pan. Bake at 450° for 15 minutes, then turn heat to 325° and bake until firm.

NO-CRUST PUMPKIN PIE

1 envelope gelatin (1 tbsp)
¼ cup cold water
3 eggs separated
⅔ cup honey
1½ cup cooked mashed pumpkin
½ cup milk
½ tsp sea salt
1 tsp cinnamon
¼ tsp nutmeg
2 tbsp honey

Soak gelatin in the cold water for 3 minutes. Beat egg yolks and combine with ⅔ cup honey, cooked pumpkin, milk, salt, cinnamon, and nutmeg in top of double boiler or in a very heavy pan over a low fire. Stir constantly until thick. Add gelatin and mix well. Beat egg whites until frothy; add 2 tbsp honey slowly. Continue beating until stiff. Pour into pumpkin mixture. Pour into well-oiled glass (9-inch) pie plate and chill several hours.

Some day, when I have a little more time between business trips, book deadlines, and lecture tours around the world, I hope to compile an entire book of Slimming Recipes That Satisfy. Until then, stay slim and be satisfied with these.

And to paraphrase what humorist Sam Levenson once said, "May there be no *pot* at the end of your rainbow."

Or anywhere else!

15

How the Beautiful People Stay Slim

Slim is a simple, uncomplicated word, the opposite of fat, which nobody wants to be.

Not so easy to define is the diverse group known as The Beautiful People of today. They may be socialites, jet-setters, the super-rich or celebrities whose names make headlines and whose faces and figures are familiar to all of us.

Or they may be none of these.

Each of us has our own conception of beauty. Mine is the one expressed by Rodin, who said, "Beauty is but the spirit breaking through the flesh."

Whatever their background, race or color, all of the Beautiful People I've known have one thing in common. None of them is fat. And though many of those included in this chapter are famous for their looks, others are more beautiful in spirit than they are in flesh.

Willie Mays is one of them. Ask his thousands of fans what they think of Willie and the answer will be unanimous "Man, he's beautiful!" The smooth coordination of his well-trained muscles is beautiful, and so is the example of discipline and good sportsmanship that he sets for a younger generation of athletes.

Sportswriter Melvin Durslag recently wrote, "Willie is, heaven help him, a product of clean living." And more than anything else, Willie's healthful way of life and balanced diet have normalized his weight and kept him firm and physically fit through the years.

Willie gets a lot of exercise, doesn't overeat, seldom drinks, and prefers lean meat and fresh vegetables to foods high in sugar and starch. He watches his weight and

173

never allows it to vary more than four pounds, going on the theory that "it's five times harder to take off twenty pounds than it is four."

If strength of character and health of body and mind are beautiful, so are the men who fight physical and emotional disabilities—the nutritionists, doctors, and psychiatrists.

Dr. Theodore Rubin, whose weight problem began during his internship, puts Willie's opinion into stronger words and warns that overweight is controllable, but not curable. "The trick is not to let it get malignant," he says, "but to get it while it's benign."

Dr. Rubin knew that he reacted to fatigue by overeating, just as most of us often do. But a busy psychiatrist can't always control the pressures that cause exhaustion. What he *could* control—and so can you—was the *type* of food he ate. He had his wife keep the refrigerator stocked with "huge quantities" of crisp, raw carrots, marinated onions, sour pickles, fresh mushrooms, celery, bean sprouts and other eat-all-you-want food.

Here is how he ate to get slim—and how he and his wife still eat to *stay* slim.

Anytime: Any of the raw, low-carbohydrate vegetables listed above, and hot tea and bouillon as desired.

Breakfast: ½ grapefruit or grapefruit juice. A three-ounce steak or canned tuna fish (water-packed or with the oil drained off) with lemon juice. No bread or toast, except now and then for company meals.

Luncheon: A large serving of scallops, shrimp, or a seafood salad or other type of fish. A low-carbohydrate vegetable or green salad, if desired, and maybe a low-calorie fruit gelatin.

Dinner: Both Dr. and Mrs. Rubin eat "a lot of veal, chicken and fish—much less beef." Steak only about once a week. No butter except when they have company. Vegetables and salad same as above. Skim milk and buttermilk are substituted for whole milk. And no desserts except fruit, low-calorie gelatin, and occasionally a pudding made with skim milk.

A Built-In Control That Prevents Overeating

Dr. Frederick Stare is another professional man who

knows from personal experience that emotional factors can trigger an eating orgy. He admits that he tends to overeat when he's worried or working under tension, so he makes a conscious effort to avoid it.

"I always eat slowly," he says.

Haven't you noticed that when you eat too fast, as nervous eaters usually do, you end up by eating too much and get up from the table feeling stuffed? Here's what Dr. Stare says about the built-in control that can prevent it if you give it a chance to work:

"It takes time for your body's blood-sugar mechanism to signal that your hunger is satisfied. If you eat slowly, within about thirty minutes your blood sugar rises; you feel satisfied before you can ask for the second helping (or dessert?) you don't really want or need. It's too bad so few of us really give this built-in safety device a chance."

Dr. Stare fights tension the same way he fights obesity— with regular daily exercise and meals high in nutrients but low in calories. Standard family meals include fish, chicken, chicken livers, lean roast beef and pot roast, occasionally hamburger and meat loaf, and steak about every two or three weeks. At least two or more vegetables, a salad and fruit round out the day's luncheon and dinner menus. No bread or butter is served, and Mrs. Stare does the cooking with vegetable oils.

"Desserts aren't much trouble," says Dr. Stare. "We just don't have them."

His daily exercise includes tennis and bicycling when he has time for them, and brisk daily walks that he *makes* time for, even on a business trip. He constantly looks for ways of getting in a fast ten- or twenty-minute walk between appointments, and to accomplish it on a crowded schedule he says, "Sometimes I damned near *run*."

MOHAMMED MOVES THE MOUNTAIN
BECAUSE OF DIET, SAYS PHYSICIAN

That was the heading of one of Pat Barham's columns in the Los Angeles *Herald-Examiner.*

The occasion was the victory of Muhammad Ali (Cassius Clay) over Jerry Quarles.

After a long absence from the ring, the heavyweight champion was quite a bit over his best fighting weight when he appeared on David Frost's television show before he went into training.

After he won the fight the question was, "How did he lose those extra pounds and get back in shape so fast?"

Two of the determining factors were Mohammed Ali's own determination and tenacity (both beautiful qualities).

The rest of the answer came from Dr. Richard You, United States Olympic Team physician, who said, "I had him on my XDR program, a balanced exercise, diet and rest program for athletes that's been Congressionally recorded. The diet consists of raw vegetables, fruits and seafood, plus lots of special vitamin supplements."

On a program like that, you too, can move mountains—mounds of excess flesh.

If laughter and talent are beautiful—and I think they are—here are two men who qualify, Jackie Gleason and Anthony Quinn.

Whatever Jackie Gleason's motivation was for losing weight, it must have been a strong one. Some say it was love. But Jackie's own explanation is psychologically sound. "There are certain periods when a person feels like losing weight," he said, "and you can do it more easily then."

There have been a lot of conflicting reports about how Jackie ate to lose sixty-one pounds, with many writers making up their own version of his diet. Some of them were so exaggerated that it isn't surprising Jackie said, "Get your weight-control advice from your doctor, not *me*."

But here, finally, is the diet Jackie Gleason used to get rid of the excess pounds standing between him and personal happiness:

How Jackie Gleason Ate to Lose Weight

Breakfast: Orange juice (small glass)
                 Two eggs (poached)
                 No bread
                 Black coffee

Luncheon: Large hamburger or small steak
                 Low-carbohydrate vegetable
                 Black coffee

Dinner: Shrimp or crabmeat appetizer
Steak (¾ lb)
Salad (with low-calorie dressing)
Two vegetables
Black coffee
No dessert (and no bread at any meal)

When it was suggested to Jackie that he could lose weight faster if he gave up liquor, he said, "I see no reason to do anything that drastic." But vermouth is high in carbohydrate, so he drank his martinis extra dry! (Let *your* conscience be your guide.)

Some years ago another formerly fat comedian, Jack E. Leonard, reduced from 360 pounds to 207. When reporters wanted to know how he did it his reply was, "By keeping my mouth shut."

Asked how much he lost, Leonard answered, "About two people."

The new Jackie Gleason lost almost "two people" without counting calories. And he did it on a much less restricted diet than Leonard's starvation program of 600 calories a day.

It was a combination of high-protein food and exercise that made the difference.

"I walked nine out of every eighteen holes on the old links," Jackie said. "I also walked a mile each morning wearing a sweat shirt and a weighted belt."

Dedicated actor Anthony Quinn purposely gained 40 pounds for the fat, balding character part he played in *The Magus.* As soon as the movie was finished Tony was eager to slim down immediately.

Lose 40 pounds *immediately?*

It can't be done. It takes a lot longer to take weight off than it does to put it on. And Tony is much too perceptive to sacrifice his health for immediacy. Luckily, he likes to walk, which is a good way to speed up any diet.

"Walking is my recreation and my exercise," he says. "I've walked in all the countries I've visited—Greece, Italy, Spain, France, Jordan, Israel—just about everywhere.

"And when I'm in Hollywood during the rain and mudslide season, I work out on an Exercycle."

The diet that worked for Tony is easy to follow and to remember. It's the *Omit-Everything-White Diet,* and here's how he describes it:

"I don't eat anything WHITE. No sugar, bread, potatoes, macaroni, cream, spaghetti—just think about everything white and omit it. That's all there is to it. In my house it takes determination, because my wife is Italian—and there goes the pasta! But the omit-everything-white diet and a lot of walking really took the extra pounds off me."

Maybe not immediately. But steadily—and with apparent safety. Except for a possible calcium shortage that could be corrected by including skim milk, buttermilk or cheese.

How a President Diets

The President of the United States a Beautiful Person?

The answer to that depends largely upon whether you're a Democrat or a Republican. But since the President's health depends upon his diet, all of us should be interested in it.

President Richard Nixon admits that he would have a weight problem if he didn't often deliberately "push back his plate" while others were still eating. According to White House chef Henry Haller, the President eats small portions of a well-balanced diet, high in energy but low in calories.

For breakfast he has fresh fruit in season or orange juice, a whole-grain cereal, usually wheat germ ("He loves wheat germ," says Haller), coffee, and a glass of milk.

Word has gotten around that the President's favorite diet luncheon is cottage cheese doused with catsup, and Haller says, "The rumor is true as far as his famous cottage cheese is concerned. He has it several days a week, but about the catsup I don't know. We prepare his cottage cheese with peaches, pineapple or other fresh fruit, and include melba toast or rye crackers and a glass of skim milk on the tray sent to his private office in the West Wing."

Sometimes instead of cottage cheese he has cold sardines or salmon (two of my favorite desk luncheons), cold roast beef, chicken, or a tuna salad.

When the Nixon family dines alone the President likes "the kind of meals we all eat at home," Swiss steak, pot roast, meat loaf, steak, a New England boiled dinner, a rib roast on Sunday, Irish stew, and fish. The President bypasses creamed dishes, and when his wife and daughter have shrimp Newburgh he eats a simple broiled fillet of sole. When they dine on chicken fricassee in cream sauce he is served a low-calorie breast of chicken with herbs. The vegetables he eats most often are those on the eat-all-you-want list, including two of his special favorites, Chinese cabbage and zucchini.

His strong sense of discipline keeps him from eating the rich desserts he likes and influences his choice of healthful, slimming foods. And whether teen-agers agree or not, discipline is beautiful.

Slimming Secrets of Beautiful Women

Here is how famous actresses, models, socialites and other Beautiful People stay slim.

Gigi Perreau: Gigi is small, so she knows it takes less food to put weight on her than it does on a larger person. "I take small portions," she says, "and never allow myself second helpings, no matter how much I enjoy a dish. It takes discipline at first, then it becomes second nature." (You see? Discipline *is* beautiful—and so are its results!)

Barbara Eden: Once a compulsive sweet-eater, Barbara admits that it took willpower and discipline (again!) to break the habit. "If I gain a few pounds they settle around my hips," she says, "so three things are necessary to keep my figure the way I like it: *willpower, exercise, and a high-protein, low-calorie diet.*"

Dinah Shore: "Maybe I'll be called a square, but I believe in staying slim and healthy through good nutrition, not fad diets," says Dinah. "If I need to lose a few pounds I eat a little less of everything, but without cutting anything out except high starches and sweets. And I always make sure that my diet is balanced, whether I'm cutting down on portions or not."

Anita Louise: "I don't consciously think of diet and exercise. I just stay active, eat well-balanced meals, avoid rich foods—and I can't remember when I last had dessert."

Julia Meade: "I just try to eat sensibly, for health and energy, and that keeps me slim. I eat a lot of Swiss chard, kale, wheat germ, brewer's yeast, yogurt, carrot juice and dandelion greens. I also try to buy things that aren't chemically grown—organic fruits and vegetables are so much better for your body."

Carol Lynley: As a teen-ager Carol nearly ruined her health with crash diets. After getting professional treatment for a troubled skin and B-12 shots for anemia, she says, "I was told to make up my own menus from a list of nutrition-rich foods that included liver, fish, chicken, lean meat, eggs, natural cheese, lots of fresh vegetables, salads, fresh fruit, milk—*but no dessert.*"

Now in her twenties, Carol still eats to stay slim, protect her health, and keep her youthful beauty.

Marjorie Lord: Some years ago Marjorie Lord played Danny Thomas' wife in his television show, *Make Room for Daddy.* After a long absence from the screen she's back playing as a grandmother in Danny's new show, *Make Room for Granddaddy.* As slim and youthful as she was when she first appeared on the screen, Marjorie tells how she stays that way:

"I do a series of push-backs. No, not push-ups—push-backs, which are harder. I push back from the table before it's time for second helpings or dessert."

Joan Crawford: Steak, liver, spinach salad and other leafy greens and tomatoes are among Joan Crawford's favorite foods. With food like that it isn't surprising that she hasn't really had a weight problem in years. And listen to what she likes for dessert: "Instead of eating dessert I eat a dill pickle. I've always liked sour things, and I found that when I was tempted to eat sweets, the opposite taste-extreme—something sour!—satisfied the craving. Now I've conditioned myself so that when others are eating fattening desserts my mouth only waters for a nice, juicy, kosher dill pickle."

Anna Maria Alberghetti: "Spaghetti and ice cream were two of my favorite foods, so of course I had a weight problem as a teen-ager. It took a lot of soul-searching and discipline to give up my special type of 'soul food,' but I finally made up my mind that being slim meant more to me than indulging myself. I gave up all starches and desserts, ate plenty of lean meat, green vegetables and fresh fruit—and lost eight pounds in three weeks!"

Angela Lansbury: Dieting has been practically a way of life for Angela since 1944, when, as a young girl, she starred in *Gaslight.* She says she's a "slow-burner" who puts on weight easily, and "bust, belly and bottom all tend to get sloppy." (Her description, not mine!) When I saw her on Broadway in *Mame* in 1966, that description didn't fit. She was trim, svelte and decidedly un-sloppy from *any* angle.

I know, because I took a good look at all of them.

Angela's lifetime eating plan is based on the *type* of food she eats rather than the *amount*, and she has found that she can lose weight faster on three small meals a day and three snacks than she can by eating one or two large meals a day. (Remember the success of Dr. Cohn's experiment with snackers in Chapter 6?)

Angela knew that she had to turn her back on desserts, bread, rice, noodles, spaghetti and all high-starch vegetables such as lima beans, corn, and dried beans and peas. Here are the foods she eats to give her "enormous energy," fill her up, slim her down and *keep* her slim:

Lean hamburger, steak, and other lean meats, chicken livers, eggs, yogurt, cheese, apples and leafy green salads. She makes her own low-calorie salad dressing with tomato, a little dry white wine, lemon juice, seasoned salt and salad herbs to taste.

"And half a grapefruit with each meal seems to have the effect of stopping the meal from staying on your fanny," is another of Angela's diet tips.

How Does a Busy Model Keep Her Lovely Figure?

Here is how three world-famous models answered the question.

Chris Noel: "My diet is simple, slimming and satisfying. It's protein foods—a lot of lean meat, but never anything fried—fresh vegetables and fruits. If I start to *feel* a pound or two heavier I cut down to smaller portions, which beats crash dieting any day. I keep very active walking to bookings, averaging several miles a day, so I don't need any other exercise."

Beverly Owen: "I eat mostly high-protein food, fresh vegetables, yogurt and salads, with as little bread, potatoes and desserts as possible. A sample of my daily menu runs like this:

"Eggs, fresh fruit or juice and coffee for breakfast.

"Yogurt for luncheon.

"Broiled meat, vegetables and green salad for dinner."

Regina Schwarz: Germany's most photographed model has been called "the new, emancipated European woman." But even an emancipated woman must discipline herself to stay slim and photogenic. Regina says that "food is a constant temptation" that she has to control. And control it she does, with almost Yogilike discipline. It takes only a single sentence to tell how she eats to stay slim:

She lives on fish, fresh vegetables, fruit and honey.

Eileen Ford: Both Eileen and her husband, Benson Ford, are weight- and cholesterol-conscious, so they also eat a lot of fish. The lovely owner of the model agency that bears her name says that she has collected "about four thousand fish and seafood recipes."

Their diet consists mainly of leafy green vegetables, salads, and all varieties of fish.

Sometimes they switch from fish to liver or chicken, but Eileen says, "We found we lost more weight eating fish than we did eating meat."

What about desserts? Her voice had a firm, disciplined ring as she answered, "You can talk yourself out of liking them!"

Jackie Onassis: Once America's beloved First Lady, now the First Lady of the International Jet Set, slender and graceful Jackie makes headlines wherever she goes. Are Jackie's secrets of slimming so costly and time-consuming that only a few can afford them? A White House physician during the Kennedy administration has the answer to that, and the simplicity of the report may surprise you.

"Jacqueline achieved her enviable figure mostly because of two facts," says Dr. Janet Travell. "(1) She is not given to excess in eating or anything else, and (2) she loves physical activity."

You know about the balance between your calorie intake and energy output, and how it can cause you to lose weight, gain weight, or stay as slim—or as fat!—as you are.

But not many of us control it as well as Jackie does.

Whether it comes from discipline or preference, she eats lightly of nonfattening foods.

Certainly Jackie is no stranger to discipline. We saw a beautiful example of it during a tragic period of her personal history—and ours.

As a chubby little girl she was fond of sweets, and as

millions of fatties can testify, it's a fondness not easily outgrown. But either Jackie outgrew it or she disciplines herself, for today she seldom touches them.

Heredity, a love of sports formed in childhood and an active participation in them set the pattern of her adult life. Her mother and father were both slender and athletic, and Jackie was put on her first horse before she was a year old.

From her school days to the present, thousands of pictures must have been published of Jackie, but have you ever seen one of her just sitting? I never have. Not even in those unauthorized pictures of her in a bikini, taken by a photographer who had no right to intrude on her privacy. She was doing a series of difficult yoga exercises that included the Lotus position, the Shoulder Stand, Plow, and yoga breathing exercises. And as anybody knows who has tried yoga exercises, they take discipline.

Most of the stories of Jackie's "diet secrets" have been highly embellished repetitions of the known facts, second-guessing, or outright fabrications.

The truth is, no embellishment is necessary, and there is nothing "secret" about them.

The two-point program stated by Dr. Travell is enough to account for Jackie's figure: *She is not given to excess in eating, and she loves physical activity.*

Jane Fonda: When Jane saw her first screen test, she says, "I left the projection room in a state of shock. I looked much too heavy, and the extra pounds had all gathered around my hips. I love bread, butter, cake and ice cream, but I stopped eating them and started on a health and reducing program. I lost fifteen pounds in three weeks on a diet of lean meat, steak, eggs, cheese, leafy greens and raw vegetables and lots of yogurt."

After her marriage to French director Roger Vadim, they lived for a while on a farm about an hour from Paris. "We grew our own fruits and vegetables and lived on natural foods, forgetting there was such a thing as junk packaged food until we returned to America. When I went into a supermarket for the first time in two years, I thought I'd never seen so many fat women in my life!" Jane's voice rose indignantly as she continued, "The market was jammed with all those fat women with big, fat fannies buying all that fattening food! I couldn't believe it!

Don't they ever get a rear view of themselves in those tight pants?"

When she's in Hollywood, Jane shops mostly in health-food stores. So slim now that she never has to diet, she likes wheat germ and honey for energy. And she still skips bread, butter and dessert and sticks to high-protein foods with lots of raw vegetables and yogurt.

Which is probably the reason she doesn't have to diet now.

For the closing advice on staying slim, it seems only fair to give the men another chance.

(Come on, girls—you *know* you always get the last word—give us a break this time! It's from only one man, and just a *few* words.)

Robert Stack: After more than thirty years in film and television pictures, how does this man manage to look as slim, handsome—and almost as youthful—as he did when he began his career in 1939?

"I've always eaten a high-protein diet," he says, "and I like health foods. I'm in an energy-burning business, so I try to have an afternoon pick-up on the set—usually orange juice spiked with honey. And I buy as much organically grown stuff as possible—lots of fresh vegetables and fruits."

At his Bel Air home he swims and plays tennis, works with weights sometimes, gets in a golf game when he has a chance, and does chin-ups and leg-ups on an exercise bar "almost every day," but doesn't follow any regular routine other than that, "except to play it by ear."

Then the man who has had "a lifelong love affair with athletics" gave this valuable advice on staying slim that everyone should follow:

"If I notice a certain part of my anatomy is beginning to sag or bulge, *I start working on it immediately*. The secret of staying in reasonably good shape is never to let your body (or your appetite?) get out of control. ... *Start taking corrective measures before it's too late.*"

No, you don't have to spend a lot of time and money to stay slim.

The Beautiful People you've just read about can afford both, but they don't find it necessary.

Staying slim is their way of life.

It can be yours, too.

16

The Eat-Your-Age Way to Stay Slim

If you're an adult, it's reasonable to assume that you've reached your final stature. You don't expect to grow any taller.

But are you still growing sideways?

Unfortunately, that's a growth that isn't self-limiting. It affects both the young and the old, and there's no age barrier or generation gap that stops it.

It's up to you whether you grow older and wiser—or older and *wider*.

Nobody else can stunt your sideways growth, and hopefully, you've already done it.

Haven't you?

If you have, you've rediscovered the joy of being slim and physically fit once more. I know. After I lost the weight I gained for my experiment it felt so great to be slim again that I paraphrased these lines of Wordsworth's to describe it:

> Of all glad words of tongue or pen,
> The gladdest are these—I'm slim again!

Come to think of it, *glad* is putting it mildly when you consider some of these rewards of positive shrinking:

You can drop something on the floor and pick it up without calling for help—to pick you up. . . .

You can give away those full skirts and wear a tight sheath. . . .

You can jog indoors without having the floors groan in protest—and without falling through them. . . .

You can wear a bikini instead of a muumuu at the beach. . . .

You can buy a smaller belt and not have to loosen it at every meal. . . .

You can sit on a sofa without leaving it rump-sprung. . . .

You can wear slacks without leaving *them* rump-sprung. . . .

You can get up out of a low-slung chair without a derrick. . . .

You begin to feel more like a Beautiful Person and less like a garbage disposal. . . .

You realize that you *are* a Beautiful Person and not a garbage disposal. . . .

You can embrace your wife or girl friend (or your husband, boy friend, or whomever) without standing sideways so your stomach won't keep you apart. . . .

You can wear new clothes that make you feel sinfully sexy. . . .

And you've gained new vitality—and virility—that makes you *feel* sinfully sexy!

Now that you're slim again you look younger, feel younger, *are* younger. Your viewpoint has changed from a looking-at-yesterday outlook to a make-way-for-tomorrow frame of mind.

What does tomorrow hold for you?

Your dieting days are over. You no longer need to reduce, but you don't want to gain back what you lost, either. You just want to maintain your weight the way it is, so you go on a maintenance diet. Ideally, it consists of more generous portions of the same high-protein, low-carbohydrate foods you ate to lose weight, plus a few extras added to it gradually. Maybe a baked potato and some whole-grain bread or cereal now and then (but not too often!). And occasionally some of the higher-carbohydrate vegetables and fruits and something sweet, but not rich (and only occasionally!).

A good maintenance diet should provide all of the essential nutrients at a low-calorie cost, equalize your daily food intake and energy output, and keep you at your normal weight the rest of your life.

But will it?

It will if you adjust your food intake or increase your

energy output every decade according to your age and way of life.

The Eat-Your-Age-and-Way-of-Life Diet

No, this isn't a new diet. Just more of the same. Or to be specific, it's the same maintenance diet, but with each passing decade you need either a little more energy output or a little less calorie intake to prevent a weight gain.

As you grow older, your dietary needs change. Not in quality, but in quantity. Your body functions more slowly, and less fuel is required to keep it running. Unless your energy output is periodically increased—which seldom happens from middle-age on—it's the diet that must gradually be scaled down.

Dr. William H. Sebrell, chairman of the NRC's food and nutrition subcommittee, warns that everyone between the ages of 35 and 55 must cut their calorie intake by 3 percent each decade or risk a weight gain that can shorten their lives.

Other experts advise a larger calorie cut for each decade. Dr. Harold W. Hermann says, "Calorie intake should be reduced about 5 percent for each ten years between 35 and 55, and 8 percent for each ten years between 55 and 75. ... The average 30-year-old woman needs about 2,200 calories daily (to maintain her weight); the average 70-year-old needs only 1,600." (My parenthetical comment.) And a man needs six to ten percent more calories than a woman does.

"But you promised us a diet that didn't require calorie counting," some of you protest, "and now you say we must cut calories by so many percentage points as we grow older. How can we tell how much to cut if we don't count the calories we eat?"

There's a way of figuring it, not quite as scientific as counting calories, but it's practical. It's a method used in various ways since Biblical times.

Food Tithing

Everybody knows what tithing is. Some of you have tithed your income, giving 10 percent to your church, a favorite charity, or some other worthy cause. Like your-self. Haven't you ever tithed for something you want, putting away 10 percent of your salary before turning the other 90 percent over to your wife? (Wives may call it "holding out," but we think of it as tithing.)

Instead of counting calories, tithe your food. Just do a quick estimate of the food on your plate and push the percentage you're supposed to tithe to one side as neatly as possible. (Nobody likes a sloppy tither!) Don't worry if your tithing measurements aren't quite accurate at first. Your scales will tell you which way they're off, and you can adjust accordingly.

If you have the clean-plate habit and can't resist eating all the food on your plate, it's a good idea to have your tithing done in the kitchen so you won't be tempted. Still, you might be able to resist temptation. It's strange, but the word "tithe" seems to have a powerful effect on people. A friend of mine who was tithing once asked his wife for a second helping of a dish he particularly liked. When she reminded him that he had some left on his plate, he said indignantly, "You know I can't eat that—it's my 5 percent tithe!"

(Saving your tithe and eating a second helping is *not* recommended.)

Another time the name "tithe" carried a lot of weight—if you'll pardon the expression!—is when you're invited out for dinner. If your hostess urges you to eat more than you should and you say, "I'm on a diet," she'll use all her wiles to get you to break it. But say, "No, thank you, I'm tithing," and not even the most persuasive hostess will insist—though some of them may think you're saving it for the needy and wrap it up in a people-bag for you.

An Automatic Weight Control for Life

Dr. Wendell Griffith, of UCLA, a member of the American Medical Association's Council on Foods and Nutrition, doesn't call it tithing, but his pattern of lifetime weight control amounts to the same thing.

"Most of us gain weight very slowly," says Dr. Griffith. "We eat perhaps 50 calories a day more than we burn. I find it easy to trim that much from my diet."

Omitting one pat of butter does it for Dr. Griffith, or

having one slice of toast for breakfast instead of two. That's usually enough to maintain his normal weight, but when it doesn't he cuts down on the overall size of his portions—like tithing a certain percent of his food calories.

"The beauty of this method," says Dr. Griffith, "is that it soon becomes a habit. Now I ask for *small* portions, even of my favorite foods, and I savor each bite. I pay attention to what I eat, and realize that I don't really want as much as I had been eating. For me—and for most people—cultivating the proper attitude toward food and eating according to your age, sex, size, and activity becomes an automatic weight control for life."

Of course there is another extreme—the men and women who get thinner and thinner with each decade that passes. They have a weight problem, too, and very little has been written about it. The same nutritious foods recommended for fatties will benefit them, but more of it, plus the healthful but high-carbohydrate foods restricted on reducing diets and the concentrated supplements I've recommended for years.

Whether you're too fat or too thin, you need the same *quality* food, so before you start your lifetime weight control by decreasing the quantity (or if you're too thin, increasing it), ask yourself these questions:

What kind of calories should be cut—or increased?

What is the overall quality of my daily meals?

Does each of them contain complete protein in sufficient amounts?

Do they contain enough unsaturated fats (such as the safflower oil in HOV) to provide the essential fatty acids?

Do they supply the vitamins, minerals, and enzymes (from raw vegetables and fruits) necessary to maintain health?

Does my diet omit processed and packaged foods that are high in calories and low in nutrients, and other foods high in starch and sugar?

Does it supply sufficient natural carbohydrates (from fresh fruits and vegetables, and when weight is stabilized, a *limited* amount of whole-grain cereal and bread) to provide the glucose that feeds the brain, supplies energy, and spares the protein necessary to build new cells and renew old ones?

If all these food elements are essential to health—and

they are!—when the decades are gaining on you and so are the pounds, where should you start tithing?

Dr. Robert Atkins, a specialist in carbohydrate metabolism and obesity control, gives his expert opinion:

"In dieting, you can either cut down caloric intake *across the board* (fats, proteins, everything) OR you can cut down carbohydrate intake (starches and sugar), and then you don't necessarily have to cut the *caloric* intake. *This is the method I strongly prefer.*" (Dr. Atkins' italics and emphasis.)

Dr. Atkins is greatly concerned over the fact that the average American diet is "overwhelmingly and inappropriately high in carbohydrates," with the median intake amounting to more than 60 percent of our diet. He has seen how our efforts to adapt to this imbalance has resulted in disorders of carbohydrate metabolism in a high percentage of the population, which is one of the major reasons for our overweight society.

"I have very bitter feelings about carbohydrates," Dr. Atkins continues. "I resent them terribly for what they do to people!"

And finally, a 2,000-year-old system of staying slim and healthy from a Greek physician, Diocles Carystos, who wrote:

"Eat your raw vegetables first of all and follow with cooked food (meat, fish or fowl) as your second course, and let fruit be the end of your meal."

It's still about the best advice I can give you for a lifetime of health and weight-control.

Why not try it?

Special Supplement

Contents:

Eat-All-You-Want Foods

These are the same low-carbohydrate hunger-savers listed in Chapter 6, repeated here for easy reference when you want something in a hurry to stave off hunger. Eat all you want of them, either lightly cooked, raw in salads, or as between-meal snacks.

artichokes, globe and	lettuce
Jerusalem	mushrooms
asparagus	mustard greens

ots
and wax

cabbage
cauliflower
celery
chard
chicory
Chinese cabbage
Chinese water chestnuts
cucumber
endive
escarole
kale

parsley
pepper, green and red
pickles
pimientos
radishes
romaine
sauerkraut, low salt, naturally
   fermented
spinach
summer squash
tampala
turnip greens
watercress
zucchini

Go-Slow Foods

For a faster weight loss, omit these relatively high-carbohydrate fruits and vegetables from your diet, or at least limit yourself to no more than one serving a week from the list until you've slimmed down. Then to *stay* slim, eat them only occasionally and in judicious quantities.

all fruit juices (except small
   amounts of grapefruit and
   tomato juice)
bananas
beets
blueberries
corn
figs
gooseberries
grapes
guavas

mangoes
parsnips
pears
peas
persimmons
potatoes (small baked or
   boiled in skin)
prunes (and other dried
   fruits)
winter squash

Go-Go Foods

(THE PROTEIN GROUP)

What can I say about the Protein Group that I haven't already told you?

These are the Go-Go foods that help you lose weight rapidly and safely and keep you from feeling like the reducer who said that his "get up and go had got up and went."

MEAT: Hamburger, steak, roast beef; liver (all kinds)

and other organ meats; veal steak, roast, cutlet and chops. Almost any lean meat EXCEPT pork, sausage, bologna and various luncheon meats with bread or cereal fillers.

FISH AND SEAFOOD: The exceptions are oysters, clams, mussels, and smoked and pickled fish.

POULTRY: Chicken, Cornish hens, turkey, and duckling, roasted, oven-fried or broiled (and *don't* eat the skin!).

EGGS: Any way except fried.

CHEESE: Farmer, pot and cottage cheese; cheddar, American, Swiss, and other natural, unprocessed cheese.

OTHER DAIRY PRODUCTS: Skim milk, buttermilk, and low-fat yogurt. (In limited amounts on restricted diets)

No-No Foods

These are the forbidden foods, off limits, *verboten*, the absolute no-no's for dieters who want to get slim—and for non-dieters who want to *stay* slim.

1. All fried foods.
2. All foods prepared in sauces and gravies.
3. All cakes, cookies, pies, pastries and other rich desserts made with ingredients I call TIF (a *T*rio of *I*nsidious *F*atteners better known as white flour, white sugar, and saturated fats).
4. Bread and crackers.
5. Candy or chocolate in *any* form.
6. Cocktails (especially the sweet ones!)
7. Cream and whipped cream.
8. Custards and puddings made with cream and sugar.
9. Doughnuts and sweet rolls (they're loaded with the menacing TIF).
10. Dried beans and peas, all kinds.
11. Fatty meats (and trim off the visible fat from all meats).
12. Gravy, cream sauces, and rich salad dressings.
13. Ice cream.
14. Jellies and jams.
15. Macaroni, noodles, spaghetti and white rice.
16. Pork and pork products (sausage and cold cuts).
17. Cream soups or thickened soups.
18. White sugar in any form.

Your Power-of-Positive-Shrinking Charts

Keeping an image in your mind of the slender, youthful person you want to be is an important factor in a reducing program. And to prevent backsliding and make the goal a reality, keep a written record of your progress to see how you're stacking up (literally—in pounds and inches!).

I. YOUR WEEKLY PROGRESS CHART

Date started **10-25-73**   Pounds overweight **43 - 47**   Desired weight **110-115**

	weight lbs.	weight loss	waist in.	hips in.	thighs in.	legs in.	arms in.	
At start of diet	157		35½	40½	24	14	12½	add 41
End of 1st week	153	4	35	40¼	24	14	12	41
(Nov. 21) 2nd week	148	5	34	39½	23¾	13¾	11¾	39¾
3rd week								
4th week								
5th week								
6th week								
7th week								
8th week								
9th week								
10th week								
11th week								
12th week								
13th week								
14th week								

II. YOUR CHEAT-AND-PENALTY CHART

Unless you have an iron will you'll probably cheat on your diet occasionally. Writing down the food you cheated on and the weight gain resulting from it may help prevent further cheating.

If that doesn't work, try to balance your cheat-food with a penalty that equalizes your energy intake and output. Long, brisk walks or extra hours of almost any vigorous exercise will do it. So will a day—or several meals—of semi-fasting.

	This Week I Cheated	Pounds Gained	My Penalty
Mon.			
Tues.			
Wed.			
Thurs.			
Fri.			
Sat.			
Sun.			

III. YOUR RESIST-AND-REWARD CHART

You've cheated a little and paid the penalty for it. Now you're sticking to your diet, refusing desserts and resisting the temptation to overeat, so you deserve a reward.

Make a list of the fattening foods you refused during the week in the *Resist* column. In the *Reward* column, write the number of pounds lost (or not gained) by your resistance. That should be reward enough, but if it isn't, treat yourself to something special. It could be new clothes in a smaller size, an appointment with a hair stylist, tickets to a play, a slimming gourmet meal, or anything you like and can afford—as long as it isn't fattening!

	This Week I Resisted	Pounds Lost	My Reward
Mon.			
Tues.			
Wed.			
Thurs.			
Fri.			
Sat.			
Sun.			

Index